CENTAURY FC
ROCK ROSE FOR PISCES

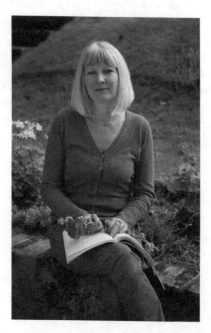

Debbie Sellwood (www.debbiesellwood.com) was born in
Surrey and now lives in a small Hampshire village, the mother
of three grown-up children. Working in the computer industry
for many years, she was very involved in the logical, rational
world until an increasing awareness in 'the bigger picture' of
life prompted her to pursue the study of astrology and seek
greater spiritual understanding of herself and others. After
gaining a diploma from the White Eagle School of Astrology
in 1999, she has worked as a consultant astrologer. Later,
she entered the field of vibrational medicine, of which the
essences are a part, and found how the two areas of study
could combine. She is Treasurer of the British Flower and
Vibrational Essences Association, and has written articles
for the astrological press, for journals covering personal
development, and for *Juno* parenting magazine.

LIMIT OF LIABILITY/DISCLAIMER OF WARRANTY

CENTAURY FOR VIRGO, ROCK ROSE FOR PISCES

*More than 400 Flower
Essences for your Zodiac Path*

Debbie Sellwood

with a foreword by Clare G. Harvey
and illustrations by Rosemary Young

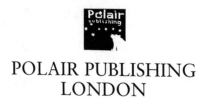

POLAIR PUBLISHING
LONDON

First published November 2007
by Polair Publishing, P O Box 34886, London W8 6YR

PERMISSIONS

I am grateful for permission to reproduce the following copyright material and quotations: To Australian Bush Flower Essences www.ausflowers.com.au and Findhorn Press, Scotland for quotations from *Australian Bush Flower Essences* and Bantam Books, Australia for *Australian Bush Flower Healing*, both by Ian White. To Living Essences of Australian Flowers www.livingessences.com.au and Australian Flower Essence Academy for quotations from *Australian Flower Essences for the 21st Century*, by Vasudeva and Kadambii Barnao. To Alaskan Essences Inc. www.alaskan-essences.com and Alaskan Flower Essence Project for quotations from *The Essence of Healing* by Steve Johnson. To Findhorn Flower Essences www.findhornessences.com and Findhorn Press, Scotland for quotations from *Findhorn Flower Essences* by Marion Leigh. To Flower Essence Society, California 0800-736-9222 www.flowersociety.com for quotations from *Flower Essence Repertory* by Patricia Kaminski and Richard Katz. To Light Heart Flower Essences www.lightheartessences.co.uk and Waterlily Books, Halesworth, UK for quotations from *Truly Divine* by Rose Titchiner. To Spirit-in-Nature Essences www.Spirit-in-Nature.com and Hay House, USA for quotations from *The Essential Flower Essence Handbook* by Lila Devi. To Pacific Essences Canada www.pacificessences.com for quotations from *Energy Medicine* by Sabina Pettitt. To Petite Fleur Essences Inc. www.aromahealthtexas.com and Paraview Press, New York, NY for quotations from *Flowers that Heal* and Herbal Health Inc. Publications, Texas for those from *The Healing Flowers*, both by Judy Griffin Ph. D. To Louise Hay and Hay House Publishers, London, for quotations from *You Can Heal Your Life*, by Louise Hay. To the Random House Group, Rushden, Northants., for quotations from *Frontiers of Health* by Dr Christine R Page. To Vega Books, 151 Freston Road, London, for quotations from *The Bodymind Workbook*, by Debbie Shapiro.

British Library Cataloguing in Publication Data
A catalogue record for this book is available from the British Library
ISBN 978-1-905398-13-3

Set in Sabon at the Publishers
Printed and bound in Great Britain
by Cambridge University Press

CONTENTS

FOREWORD by Clare G. Harvey   9
ACKNOWLEDGMENTS   10

INTRODUCTION   11
All about flower essences   13
   1. *What are they?*   13
   2. *How are they made?*   14
   3. *How do they work?*   15
   4. *How can they help?*   18
   5. *How to take flower essences*   20
   6. *What can be expected when*
     taking essences?   21
Selecting essences for yourself   23
   1. *The body–mind message*   23
   2. *Astrology's correspondence with the*
     body–mind message   24
   3. *The twelve constitutional types*   27

1   THE ARIES OUTLOOK ON LIFE AND
      HEALTH (March 21–April 20)   29
   Constitution   29
   Healing and self-development for Aries subjects   30
   Suggested essences for Aries subjects 33
     Resolving possible personality imbalances   33
     Balancing Arian energy   37
     Relating and communicating 41
     Resolving possible physical imbalances   47

2   THE TAURUS OUTLOOK ON LIFE AND
      HEALTH (April 20–May 21)   49
   Constitution   49
   Healing and self-development for Taureans   50
   Suggested essences for Taureans   53

Resolving possible personality imbalances 53
Balancing Taurean energy 58
Relating and communicating 63
Resolving possible physical imbalances 66

3 THE GEMINI OUTLOOK ON LIFE AND HEALTH
(May 21–June 22) 69
Constitution 69
Healing and self-development for Geminians 70
Suggested essences for Geminians 72
Resolving possible personality imbalances 72
Balancing Gemini energy 77
Relating and communicating 82
Resolving possible physical imbalances 87

4 THE CANCER OUTLOOK ON LIFE AND HEALTH
(June 22–July 23) 90
Constitution 90
Healing and self-development for Cancerians 91
Suggested essences for Cancerians 94
Resolving possible personality imbalances 94
Balancing Cancerian energy 98
Relating and communicating 103
Resolving possible physical imbalances 108

5 THE LEO OUTLOOK ON LIFE AND HEALTH
(July 23–August 23) 110
Constitution 110
Healing and self-development for Leos 111
Suggested essences for Leos 113
Resolving possible personality imbalances 113
Balancing Leo energy 118
Relating and communicating 123
Resolving possible physical imbalances 127

6 THE VIRGO OUTLOOK ON LIFE AND HEALTH
(August 23–September 23) 130
Constitution 130
Healing and self-development for Virgoans 131

Suggested essences for Virgoans — 134
Resolving possible personality imbalances — 134
Balancing Virgoan energy — 139
Relating and communicating — 143
Resolving possible physical imbalances — 147

7 THE LIBRA OUTLOOK ON LIFE AND HEALTH
 (September 23–October 24) — 150
Constitution — 150
Healing and self-development for Librans — 151
Suggested essences for Librans — 154
Resolving possible personality imbalances — 154
Balancing Libran energy — 158
Relating and communicating — 162
Resolving possible physical imbalances — 167

8 THE SCORPIO OUTLOOK ON LIFE AND
 HEALTH (October 24–November 22) — 169
Constitution — 169
Healing and self-development for Scorpios — 170
Suggested essences for Scorpios — 172
Resolving possible personality imbalances — 172
Balancing Scorpio energy — 178
Relating and communicating — 182
Resolving possible physical imbalances — 186

9 THE SAGITTARIUS OUTLOOK ON LIFE AND
 HEALTH (November 22–December 22) — 189
Constitution — 189
Healing and self-development for Sagittarians — 190
Suggested essences for Sagittarians — 192
Resolving possible personality imbalances — 192
Balancing Sagittarian energy — 196
Relating and communicating — 201
Resolving possible physical imbalances — 206

10 THE CAPRICORN OUTLOOK ON LIFE AND
 HEALTH (December 22–January 21) — 208
Constitution — 208

Healing and self-development for Capricornians   210
Suggested essences for Capricornians   212
    Resolving possible personality imbalances   212
    Balancing Capricorn energy   217
    Relating and communicating   221
    Resolving possible physical imbalances   225

11   THE AQUARIUS OUTLOOK ON LIFE AND
     HEALTH (January 21–February 19)   228
Constitution   228
Healing and self-development for Aquarians   230
Suggested essences for Aquarians   232
    Resolving possible personality imbalances   232
    Balancing Aquarian energy   237
    Relating and communicating   241
    Resolving possible physical imbalances   245

12   THE PISCES OUTLOOK ON LIFE AND HEALTH
     (February 19–March 21)   248
Constitution   248
Healing and self-development for Pisceans   249
Suggested essences for Pisceans   251
    Resolving possible personality imbalances   251
    Balancing Piscean energy   256
    Relating and communicating   261
    Resolving possible physical imbalances   265

EPILOGUE: THE ESSENCE OF MASTERING
     OUR LIVES   268

APPENDICES   269
    1. *Bibliography and reading list*   269
    2. *The 'Purely Essences' range*   270
    3. *Index by emotions and states of mind*   271
    4. *Essence distributors*   283
    5. *Essence producers*   284
    6. *Index of essences*   285

FOREWORD

HUMANKIND has always sought to understand itself in greater depth.

There is no double that ancient man was more in touch with his environment, and it is clear from what is known from the Egyptian or Tibetan civilizations that they closely observed the movements of the sun, moon, stars and planets. Man's desire to comprehend his essential nature as well as his relationship to and place within the world and the universe led man to see how profoundly he was influenced and shaped by it. Astrology grew out of this insight and vision of the interconnectedness of all life.

I am delighted to be able to recommend the first comprehensive in-depth study on the transformational effect of flower essences, not only in strengthening our astrological makeup but also as tools to evolve beyond the constraints of our star signs.

Debbie has given practical solutions to comprehending our individual body/mind messages, specially our negative ones, and by researching the appropriate remedies as aids for self-healing and re-empowerment has given us a key to self-mastery. This development of our inner potential encourages us to discover where our true spiritual purpose lies—an important discovery at this stage of the planet's evolution when mankind's future hangs in the balance.

Clare G Harvey
September 2007

Author, Teacher and International Flower Remedy Expert at Clinic for Complementary and Integrated Medicine in Upper Harley Street

ACKNOWLEDGMENTS

I SHOULD like to give my thanks to Simon Bentley who many years ago patiently instructed and encouraged me to develop my skills as an astrologer while I completed the courses of the White Eagle Lodge School of Astrology.

Clare Harvey's course in Vibrational Medicine, a journey and experience in itself, broadened my awareness and opened my mind to the potential of flower essences as a form of healing, empowerment and much more. To her my thanks and also in providing the foreword for this book. In addition my thanks go to Julian Barnard for providing the supportive comments.

My dream of combining both subjects most close to my heart into a book has been enabled by Colum Hayward of Polair Publishing. To him I give my thanks for bringing this book into being. I also thank Rosemary Young, whose drawings grace the chapter openings, and Sandra Richardson, who kindly contributed the flower illustrations on the cover.

I also give thanks for the encouragement and support received from my family and friends and the insights gained through my clients and their healing journeys.

*I should like to dedicate this book
to Brian, Kelly, Ross and Keira, the stars in
my life and the essence of my being!*

INTRODUCTION

'That which is looked upon by one generation as the apex of human knowledge is often considered an absurdity by the next, and that which is regarded as a superstition in one century, may form the basis of science for the following one.'
PARACELSUS

CONSIDERED by many to be the 'medicine' of the future, vibrational essences—most commonly known as flower essences, a term I shall use as shorthand for them all—are making a significant contribution to humanity. The gift they bring from nature is life-healing, life-enhancing, and life-affirming. Their actions have a far-reaching implication for humanity and for the world, not just physically, mentally and emotionally but in the spiritual upliftment of consciousness.

With this in mind, CENTAURY FOR VIRGO, ROCK ROSE FOR PISCES has been written to bring the benefits of flower essences to a wider audience, to make the choice of right essence easier, and to enhance the potential the remedies have for the unfoldment of total being. It is a comprehensive reference to the healing and transformational qualities of hundreds of flower, gem and environmental essences from all over the world. The book is arranged as a practical guide to enable you to use astrology as your diagnostic type. Astrology can help you to recognize any weak points, imbalances or qualities in your personality that you may wish to change, heal, transform or improve. Through an analysis of each of the twelve astrological 'types', the typical challenges and conflicts (mentally, emotionally and physically) that may be presented to an individual on life's journey are highlighted, along with the appropriate flower essences to overcome and handle these experiences and the associated states of mind. The book is also, of course, intended for practitioners.

Essences awaken certain qualities within the human psyche by touching the mental, emotional and spiritual aspects of our being; they address the whole person. They restore, support, encourage, awaken, strengthen and empower, thus gently bringing us in tune with our true selves, raising our spiritual awareness and enabling balance and harmony to be found within. Along with this goes improved understanding of self and self-development on an inner level, which in turn encourages the positive aspects of our personalities to shine forth more easily, and brings an increased sense of wellbeing on many levels. Thus the essences help to remove the seeds of discontent, dissatisfaction or unhappiness, which can contribute to illness. They can eventually result in improvements in physical health and in many cases resolve contributory factors so that illness does not manifest. Note that where such improvements are suggested in the text, this usually follows the resolution of other issues on a more subtle level (see pp. 21–23). Therefore, these essences do not work like prescription medicines, and should not replace them. Always consult your doctor if you suspect illness.

The key messages of this book are self-understanding and self-responsibility. If you wish to improve wellbeing in any aspect of your life and are prepared to embark upon your own journey of self-awareness and self-development, then CENTAURY FOR VIRGO, ROCK ROSE FOR PISCES can assist you in the first instance by helping you identify areas of imbalance or vulnerability, and then by suggesting appropriate essences. Alternatively you may wish to concentrate on personal or spiritual growth. If you are a therapist, you may want to utilize this book to assist others.

The twelve chapters of this book, one for each astrological sign, link suitable essences to zodiacal 'constitutional types'. Every section also contains insights into the spiritual lesson appropriate for a zodiac sign (see below, p. 25).* This perspective provides valuable understanding into our own special path in life. Having awareness of this lesson usually confirms what life has been trying to tell us anyway; we may even have already been naturally gravitating toward embracing it. Awareness of our mission enables us to position ourselves favourably, so that we can consciously direct our energy and act more purposefully, which in due course affords a sense of fulfilment and can have a direct and positive effect on our attitude and health. Remember that you can use CENTAURY FOR VIRGO, ROCK ROSE FOR PISCES as a workbook; it is intended to stay with you as a helper, not just to be used when you have an ailment!

ALL ABOUT FLOWER ESSENCES

1. WHAT ARE THEY?

FLOWER essences, said to be used by ancient civilizations, were reintroduced in more recent times by Dr Edward Bach in the 1930s. He is the father of modern-day vibrational essences, and his beliefs and theories form the basis of our understanding of how they work.

These natural remedies are made by using the energy contained in flowers and plants. Produced in liquid form, they are taken by drops under the tongue or in water. Dr Bach, when developing these remedies, recognized the link between stress, emotions and illness; his essences (along with essence ranges by other producers) help to improve our wellbeing by making actual transitions in our emotions. They do not treat physical illness directly, but rather the negative

*Note that the dates given for the astrological signs are typical for the present time. They do vary slightly from year to year, so if you are in doubt about yours because it is on the 'cusp', consult a relable astrologer. The phrase 'constitutional types' is not used here in the homeopathic sense of the word.

thoughts, feelings or inner disharmony that may manifest as physical problems. In resolving personality imbalances, they provide a gentle, holistic way of healing.

Flower essences form part of a system of vibrational healing, which sees human beings consisting of complex, multidimensional energy fields that orchestrate and organize the physical body. Vibrational healing is based on the idea that everything in the universe emits its own unique energy frequency; I believe it is also true of the physical body, which radiates its own distinct energy-signature. The vibrating, subtle-energy fields are linked with one's emotions and feelings and their condition is vital to the overall balance of one's psyche and physical health. Flower essences have the ability to influence these fields if imbalance occurs, thus restoring harmony, mentally, emotionally, spiritually and often physically. This concept is further explained in the section 'How do they work?' (p. 15).

Since Dr Bach produced his range of thirty-eight flower essences, this field has blossomed, with many producers from all over the world now creating their own ranges. In addition to essences made from flowers, essences are also created using crystals, gems, and other natural resources. This book incorporates many of these essences, including essences made from the energy of sea creatures. It should be noted that no harm is ever inflicted upon any sea creature in the making of the essences covered in this book.

2. HOW ARE THEY MADE?

Essences contain the energetic pattern of plants, crystals, gems and other sources of the natural world. Generally, when essences are made the physical constituents of a flower (or such) are not used*, only the essential energy that is found within it. This energy is captured in water and along

*Some essences are an exception to this, such as a few from the Bach range. So too is The Petite Fleur range made by Judy Griffin, a herbalist who uses the lipoic acid produced by flowers in her range of essences.

with an antibacterial preservative such as brandy it is transferred into bottles. It may seem far-fetched that water can hold an energetic pattern in this way, but how it can has now been demonstrated by the experiments of Dr Masaru Emoto. His books, MESSAGES FROM WATER, provide further information on the ability of water to retain a memory, a theory first explored by a French scientist, Jacques Benveniste, who experimented with an antibody diluted in water. This solution was further diluted until the chance that a single molecule of antibody being left was very small. However, tests for properties related to the presence of the antibody proved positive.

Only undamaged flowers, usually from wild unspoilt places in nature, grown without pesticides or fertilizers, are used. Ideally, these would be flowers that are just coming into bloom—when their energy is most potent. In making their essences, the vast majority of producers do so using a sun-infusion of blossoms in a bowl of water. The 'Sun method' used by the producers of the Healing Herbs range of Bach flower essences is described in detail in a book, THE HEALING HERBS OF EDWARD BACH, by Julian and Martine Barnard. However, some producers, very aware of conservation concerns, are now exploring alternative methods of capturing the energy of flowers without removing the blooms. As might be expected, most producers are gifted and intuitive people with a huge respect and love for flowers and other elements of nature, and special rapport with them. In most cases they have an understanding of nature that is beyond the capacity of the average person.

3. HOW DO THEY WORK?

Fully to appreciate how essences work, it is necessary to have an understanding of the non-physical parts of one's anatomy. All life-forms vibrate at an energetic level, and it is at the 'subtle energetic levels of our being' that flower essences gently work—by resonating against imbalances that may occur at these levels. Flower essences work indirectly on the physical body by influencing the subtle energy-structures that make up our total being. Their effect on the energy bodies, chakras, *nadis* and acupuncture meridians (a description of all these follows) modifies not only the life-force energy—*prana* or *qi*—which flows into the body, but also our consciousness, which ultimately affects the physical body. Working at a vibratory level, they restore, bring into alignment and balance these subtle elements. Nature seems to have provided a flower for almost every human condition or state of being, so when the vibratory frequency of an (ingested) essence resonates with an area of imbalance in a person, at any level, a 'frequency tuning' takes place. Thus balance is restored to all the higher energetic systems that ultimately influence the various cellular patterns in the physical body.

Subtle bodies

We are more than just our physical body and, as I suggested earlier, all of us consist of complex, multi-dimensional, energy fields. They are also known as subtle bodies or energy bodies. There are considered to be seven such bodies, briefly described below, and although they are separate, they are interconnected and function as a whole. Variations on the interpretation of the bodies (and the other aspects of the subtle anatomy that follow) may vary according to certain different philosophies and schools of thought.

The **Etheric** body, a replica of the physical body containing all the same physical organs, maintains the balance between the physical body and the subtle bodies.

The **Emotional body** provides a sense of emotional stability and security when balanced.

The **Mental body** enables people to think clearly and rationally when in balance.

The **Astral body** contains the total accumulation of the

personality and past-life experiences. When balanced, it enables an individual to have an intuitive understanding of events.

The **Causal body** is the doorway to higher consciousness and a link to collective consciousness.

The **Soul body** holds our spiritual essence.

The **Spiritual Body** holds our basic energetic imprint, a combination of the physical and subtle anatomy.

The chakra system

The chakras, the description of which comes down to us from the earliest Indian wisdom traditions, are situated more or less along the length of the spine but located just outside the physical body, are connected to both the meridian system and the subtle bodies. They are linked with the endocrine glands and the nerve centres in the spine. These energy centres are concerned with receiving, assimilating and transmitting higher energies into a form that the body can use. It is the *nadis* ('petals of the chakras'), linked to the nervous system, that distribute the energy of the chakras throughout the physical body. The seven main chakras (there are many more), their functions and possible areas of imbalance are described very briefly below.

The **Base Chakra**, situated at the base of the spine, is associated with identity, security, safety, survival and energy. Imbalances can manifest in foot and leg problems, structural problems, lower-back pain, constipation, arthritis and blood pressure problems.

The **Sacral Chakra**, situated just below the navel, is associated with the ability to use one's own power and creativity. Imbalances can manifest as sexual, reproductive, urinary or lower-back problems.

The **Solar Plexus Chakra**, situated just above the navel, is associated with the ego, self-esteem and emotions. Imbalances can manifest as stomach, digestive and intestinal problems.

The **Heart Chakra**, situated in the centre of the chest, is associated with self-love, compassion and universal goodwill. Imbalances can manifest as heart, circulatory, lung and respiratory problems.

The **Throat Chakra**, situated in the throat area, is associated with will, self-expression and communication. Imbalances can manifest as problems with the throat, neck, shoulders or arms, or are associated with the thyroid, parathyroid, lymph or immune system.

The **Third Eye** or **Brow Chakra**, situated in the centre of the forehead, is associated with perception, imagination and intuition. Imbalances can manifest as nervous problems, as sinusitis, or as ear and eye problems.

The **Crown Chakra**, situated at the crown of the head, is associated with consciousness, wisdom, self-awareness, spirituality and unity with all things. Imbalances can manifest as migraine headaches, epilepsy, depression and an inability to face reality.

Acupuncture Meridians

According to the teachings of Traditional Chinese Medicine, the meridian system consists of a network of channels, which spread as an intricate web throughout the body, providing a connection between the physical body and the subtle energy surrounding it. These interconnected electrical pathways conduct the vital energy, in a way analogous to what in the Indian system are called the *nadis* and chakras, to all the organs and areas of the physical body.

4. HOW CAN THEY HELP?

It is no coincidence that the knowledge about flower essences has resurfaced at this time of immense change, restlessness and exceptional trauma in the earth's history. Humanity's current progression towards a more enlightened state can certainly be accelerated if we take advantage of vibrational essences to expand our awareness and lighten our physical vibration.

Their gentle energy can offer us relief and protection against both the pressured and anxious times in which we live, and the stress of toxins in the environment. They offer support if you are troubled, confused or worried; they increase awareness, and thus the ability to consider other possibilities and to see things from another perspective. If you need to develop resilience to stress, or courage and strength to deal with challenges and trials, then they can assist. When you are physically scattered and thrown about after shock, distress and despair, they bring together, restore and integrate the aspects of your being. They help you to handle and balance areas of your life when you are ill at ease or vulnerable, and they can also aid you in releasing the past and adjusting to new circumstances or situations.

With the support of flower essences, you can make the best of yourself by healing, resolving, restoring, developing, encouraging, uplifting and enhancing certain aspects of your personality. Over a period of time, essences can bring you in tune with your true self and help you to fulfil your promise and reach your potential.

Lastly, they provide a natural, simple and effective way of healing, but one that does not interfere with or adversely affect conventional medicines or homeopathic remedies. Safe for children, they can also be used effectively with animals and plants. Essences however do not replace proper medical attention or a proper healthcare or exercise regime. Healing can take place on many levels, and in some situations the expected outcome may not always be apparent on the surface. Please see pp. 21–23 for more about this.

Just a few of the ways in which essences can assist....

⋏ *in releasing shock, trauma and upsets from your past*

⋏ *in improving self-confidence, self-worth or self-acceptance*

⋏ *in breaking down resistance to change, relieving anxiety and proneness to negative thinking, depression or sadness*

⋏ *in fulfilling your true potential, even if this involves a change from what you are doing*

⋏ *in restoring satisfaction in aspects of your personal relationships*

⋏ *in finding inner strength to face major change, challenges or problems*

⋏ *in bringing inner guidance or greater clarity around particular issues*

⋏ *in unfolding spiritual awareness or wanting to understand your higher purpose*

⋏ *in helping you let go old resentments, hurts and traumas*

⋏ *in bringing improvement in a physical condition (though essences do not work directly on the physical body but on the emotional/mental attitudes that are believed to contribute toward illness)*

⋏ *in restoring vitality following a period of illness, accident, overwork or stress*

⋏ *in unblocking creativity and dispelling apathy.*

5. HOW TO TAKE FLOWER ESSENCES

After consulting the section in the appropriate Sun-sign chapter on 'Selecting Essences for Yourself', use your intuition (sometimes known as the sixth sense) to be guided into which essence, or couple of essences, are suitable for you. The ones that you are instinctively drawn to are likely to be the ones you need. In this you may be helped first by looking at the headings outlined in black, and then at the hints italicized in the left-hand column. It is quite appropriate to select more than one essence to take at a time, if you are working on a couple of issues or conditions. Avoid attempting to resolve too many issues at once, as this can complicate things and make it difficult to observe your reaction or response (no more than half a dozen essences are advised to be taken at a time). Keep in mind that essences work to restore balance generally, so the effects of taking one essence may resolve or heal something else on another level, which was not expected. It is impossible to overdose on essences. If you inadvertently choose an essence that you do not need, then it will simply have no effect.

When a bottle of flower essence is purchased* it is in a concentrated form and is known as a 'stock bottle'. Take your essence according to the instructions on the bottle. If you are taking several essences (from any range), then it is quite appropriate to make up your own personal combination by diluting them (which does not reduce their potency) into an empty bottle. This is known as a 'dosage bottle'. To do so, take a clean dropper bottle of about 30ml (obtained from a chemist) and add 25% brandy or vodka as a preservative (when alcohol is not suitable, substitute apple cider vinegar or vegetable glycerine). Add 2 to 3 drops of each of your selected essences† (from any essence range) and fill the bottle with spring water. Take 7 drops morning and night until the bottle is finished. Keep your bottle away from sunlight, electrical appliances and chemicals. One of the most important things about taking essences is that you should do so consistently for them to be effective. Generally, essences are taken orally, although they can be used topically, in the bath or via a misting bottle.

6. WHAT CAN BE EXPECTED WHEN TAKING ESSENCES?

Some people respond quickly, after taking essences for only a few days or weeks, while others may require essences for many months or even years in order to resolve emotional

*A complete list of essence producers is given in the appendices to this book, together with a number of distributors.

†Some producers now sell 'dosage bottles', so if you are making a dosage bottle yourself then be sure to use essences from 'stock' bottles.

worries, release negative thinking or improve physical conditions. Generally, people find that the longer they have had an illness or felt a certain way, then the longer it will take to bring about new balance.

Flower essences do not work instant magic (although many people can experience quick results). Healing (on any level) often requires persistence and can be gradual, particularly where the issues are deep-seated. This is in contrast to the expectation in today's society, where instant relief is promised by many medicines and indeed expected from them (but frequently has only temporary effect, as it may not resolve the heart of the problem). Everyone's response is unique, and everyone's healing capacity is individual—so be patient. Healing is most often part of a bigger picture and unexpected improvements or changes can occur in other areas, so it pays to be observant and informally monitor your feelings while taking a course of essences. For some people, the result of taking essences can be compared with the metaphor of 'peeling an onion'. After first taking an essence, an issue may be presented in our consciousness that we may or may not have previously been aware of. This may follow the resolution of the original issue, or the current issue may need to be resolved as a prerequisite to sorting the original issue. Subsequent layers may reveal themselves and require additional essences. Complex conditions may require the expertise of a flower essence practitioner, and it is advisable to seek one through the assistance of a professional body, such as The British Flower and Vibrational Essence Association (www.bfvea.com), which has a list of practitioners on its website.

Some people find the qualities of essences so subtle that they do not think there has been any change within themselves after taking them. It is not until they reflect (or others remind them) upon how they were, or how they felt and behaved previously, that they recognize a difference. You do not have to believe that essences will work for them to do so, but it does help to be receptive and open to them.

Although not everyone experiences this, flower essences can sometimes provoke a 'healing crisis' during the first few days of taking them. This can be experienced emotionally. We may become aware of strong feelings, and may actually display irritation, anger or crying. Or physically, where a reaction occurs as the body detoxifies, there may be, for example, a skin rash, pimples or chest congestion. If there is already a physical condition present, it may worsen before getting better. Flower essences often work in this manner, presenting one with a physical manifestation of how certain issues are impacting on one's life and need to be resolved.

However, essences can be used for other reasons than improving a certain state of mind or condition, such as to provide a self-help means to personal empowerment, self-development and increased self-awareness.

SELECTING ESSENCES FOR YOURSELF

There are many thousands of essences from all over the world to choose from. One of the intentions of this book is to simplify the selection process by relating the healing and empowering qualities of the most widely available of these essences to the constitutional types of the twelve astrological signs.

1. THE BODY–MIND MESSAGE

'Physicians, when the cause of disease is discovered, consider that the cure is discovered'. CICERO

Science now recognizes that our feelings and emotions can profoundly affect our physical health. Emotions produce hormones that travel around the body and bring changes physically, in accordance with our emotional state. The work of Dr Candace Pert, published as MOLECULES OF EMOTION, brings a scientific approach to understanding how the mind and the body work together. In her capacity as a neuroscientist, and after decades of research, she is able to demonstrate that when we have an emotion, it shows up in the body as a pattern of peptides (chemical messengers) which link to appropriate receptors (receivers of these messages) in various organs and muscles of the body and affect their function, and produce a reaction. In other words, you are what you think; you create your own reality. Change your thinking and you change your life. Dr Pert's findings emphasize just how important it is to take responsibility for ourselves, and how a positive attitude is crucial in maintaining wellbeing and health.

2. ASTROLOGY'S CORRESPONDENCES WITH THE BODY–MIND MESSAGE

Astrology provides a tool by which you can become aware of the traits associated with your Sun-sign, ones which if they manifest strongly may positively or adversely affect your health and wellbeing. We all possess certain qualities or failings that greatly influence our conduct, our relationships with others and ultimately our wellbeing, although we can often be unconscious of them. We can unconsciously act out patterns of behaviour or habits that are not always in our best interest and can be detrimental to our health, not to mention happiness. Sometimes this occurs at difficult times in our life, through stress or illness. Just through the general knocks of life we can become conditioned to behaving in a negative way. When these unhelpful traits of our personality manifest, in turn they can undermine our health.

Although everybody's health legacy is unique, astrology

*Knowledge of our Sun-sign can only give a general picture of our attitude to life and the factors influencing our health. A qualified astrologer can provide considerably more information when analyzing an individual's birth chart. An astrologer who is also medically qualified can add further depth into an individual's state of health.

is based on the belief that every one of us is influenced by a certain combination of planets at the time of our birth*. This book only takes into account the position of the Sun on the day of your birth, but shows that by understanding the relationship between your Sun-sign and the physical body you can gain a vital perspective on your health. If you know what sign the Moon was in or what your Ascendant (rising sign) was at the time of your birth, then it can be helpful to read about those zodiacal signs also. The Moon gives an indication of your emotional disposition and how you feel and respond, both to events and other people. The Ascendant shows the manner in which you portray the many aspects of your character. Taking all three of these into consideration gives you the key factors in determining your overall personality. These days, information about your birthchart can be obtained from many different astrological sites on the internet if you know your time of birth as well as the day.

The notes at the start of each chapter in this book identify each Sun sign by its element—earth, fire, air and water. These elements, along with the 'quality' of the sign—cardinal, fixed or mutable—are what give it its character. From these indicators are derived the overriding 'soul-lesson' for the individual born under that sign, for the duration of its incarnation. This concept of soul-lessons is a generally-used tool in esoteric astrology, for understanding our mission not only brings into focus which area of life our lesson lies in, but it enables us to position ourselves advantageously.

The lesson that fire signs (Aries, Leo and Sagittarius) are learning is 'Love'. This may be self-love, respect for one's own being, or love for others (interpreted literally or generally in the form of selfless dedication to an association or a cause).

The lesson that earth signs (Taurus, Virgo and Capricorn) are learning is 'service'. This means identifying in which direction or capacity (according to your abilities), you can provide assistance and help to others or perhaps an organization.

The lesson that air signs (Gemini, Libra and Aquarius) are

learning is 'brotherhood'. Through understanding the needs of others, these people can bring them fellowship, care and companionship.

The lesson water signs (Cancer, Scorpio and Pisces) are learning is 'peace'. The emphasis here is in rising about the grip of the emotional level and finding a deep inner core upon which you can tackle the ups and downs of life.

A detailed description of all these lessons can be found in Joan Hodgson's books ASTROLOGY THE SACRED SCIENCE and WISDOM IN THE STARS.

The correspondences between the Sun-sign and the body were common knowledge centuries ago, when medicine was not practised without expertise in astrology. Astrology provides us with useful insights into the weak areas of the body and those areas that are potentially vulnerable if we become out of balance. That may be simply because we are subject to the strain of modern living, but it may be because we deny or ignore certain aspects of ourselves. The body has its own wisdom, and much can be learnt by paying attention to what it seems to be telling us. In this respect, books by Debbie Shapiro (THE BODYMIND WORKBOOK) and Louise Hay (YOU CAN HEAL YOUR LIFE) are insightful in discerning the messages behind physical disorders. Our emotional state is not just confined to our thoughts but affects our whole body; the mind is intimately linked with the workings of the body. If we can 'create our own illnesses', we also have the ability to take steps to avoid such problems arising. Astrology provides a means by which to understand ourselves, while flower essences play a valuable part in helping us maintain a positive, life-affirming attitude to life, one which in turn positively influences health and wellbeing.

This book is a general guide, and only potential weaknesses and likely illnesses are indicated. While you may recognize your weak spots, it does not mean that the illnesses associated with each sign will necessarily manifest. It is not until an accumulation of certain factors comes together that illness becomes probable, unless of course it is of a genetic origin. Equally, the health problems associated with each sign are not exclusive to that sign. Never ignore symptoms simply because they are not associated with your sign.

3. THE TWELVE CONSTITUTIONAL TYPES

Wonderful people that we all are, inevitably we are not perfect! Please bear in mind when reading the chapter on your Sun-sign that the purpose of this book is simply to highlight possible personality imbalances and suggest the appropriate essences to deal with them. Regrettably, the objective is not to elaborate on all the positive points, wonderful characteristics and glorious qualities of each of the twelve signs, nice though that would be!

It is important to remember the law of balance that operates in astrology. For example, if your Sun-sign is the first sign in the zodiac, Aries, then you may share some of the characteristics of your opposite sign, the seventh sign, Libra, including potentially vulnerable areas of the body. Your opposite sign is indicated at the start of each section.

It should be noted that the essences suggested for each sign are a guide only, and it does not mean that they are exclusive to that sign. For instance, *Impatiens* essence is suggested for Aries, who typically has a tendency for impatience. It is quite appropriate for anyone wanting to temper impatience, regardless of their astrological sign. When you have selected an essence, look it up in the index at the back of the book. Each name will be followed by initial letters such as AB, PF, etc. When consulting the producer or distributor index, AB (for example) will indicate that this essence is one from the Australian Bush range.

In a few cases throughout this book, a distinction is made between flower essences with the same name but from different producers. Flowers grown in one part of the world (by one producer) and under certain conditions can have slightly different characteristics from flowers growing somewhere else under different conditions (and grown by another producer). Aside from reading the chapter about your own Sun-sign, you may wish to consult—at the back of the book—the index of flower essences arranged by state of mind or emotion.

The descriptions of all essences provided in this book are not exhaustive. Further details of each can be acquired in each flower essence producer's book of their own range, which is listed in the bibliography. In the text, I have avoided endless repetition by referring to these books by their author's name only; look to the bibliography for details of the book concerned. Ian White and Judy Griffin each have two published books and I have distinguished between them with their initials. It should be noted that the description of each essence in this book is written from the perspective of the author's own experience of these essences and that of her clients, and is then in addition supported by producers' literature.

Go ahead, check out your chapter, take responsibility and be as honest as you can about yourself and then....

Become the best possible 'you' with flower essences!

1. THE ARIES OUTLOOK ON LIFE AND HEALTH

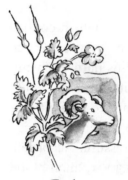

Aries

March 21–April 20

Quality & element: Cardinal Fire

Ruler: Mars

Opposite sign: Libra

Soul-lesson: Love

CONSTITUTION

THE ASTROLOGICAL symbol for Aries the Ram shows the horns and depicts the upward, thrusting, initiating energy so typical of Aries. This huge amount of physical energy needs a channel, otherwise the Aries subject can experience frustration, impatience or anger. Equally, Aries people need to watch lest their passionate and headstrong manner pushes them too hard and wears them out. Aries personalities are warm, enthusiastic, energetic and highly-motivated; others find them stimulating, inspiring and encouraging—but they can be intolerant and impetuous at times! Not afraid to take a risk, activate plans or make the first move, they usually want to take charge and often possess leadership qualities. Their sign being identified with the astrological quality known as cardinality means that they are good with 'starting energies'— instigating projects and ventures. However, they can often lose interest when their curiosity is fired by something else that brings them a new challenge.

Implications for health

The head and face are ruled by Aries. Under pressure, this can externalize as headaches or discomfort in the scalp or jaw, and as migraines, neuralgia, sinusitis or other painful conditions of the face.

Although an Aries needs new opportunities and stimulating

circumstances in which to channel his or her energies, the impulsive nature of the sign can make it all too easy for Aries people to misspend these energies, and this sometimes results in tension or discontent. If their keenness gets the better of them, it can turn to impatience—in which case they need to guard against accidents, especially burns, cuts and blows, particularly to the head and face. It is beneficial for them to learn to control and regulate their expenditure of 'headstrong' energy so as to avoid going 'headfirst' into things without thinking.

Aries is also linked to the adrenal glands, which control the flow of adrenaline in the body. If the Arian approach to life is in overdrive, then too much of this natural chemical can be produced, which can be debilitating and depleting, leaving them exhausted. Their tendency to be a bit hot-headed can mean that they are quick to anger, which can be a contributory factor to high blood pressure. According to Debbie Shapiro, in THE BODYMIND WORKBOOK, 'high blood pressure indicates a boiling, a rising of emotion, maybe anger or hurt, in relation to love'. She also attributes it to 'nervousness and anxiety giving rise to panic—a fear that the love in one's life is not dependable'. This is particularly interesting in the light of the soul-lesson of Aries, which is love (there is more on this under 'the spirit' in the next section, p. 32). It is also in the interest of Aries people to look after other areas of the face such as the teeth and eyes.

☞ For the Soul-lessons, see pp. 13 & 25

HEALING AND SELF-DEVELOPMENT FOR ARIES SUBJECTS

The mind

If you are an Aries, you can be so eager to 'do' in the outside world that you do not always take enough time out to develop your inner strengths. The expectation, particularly for the young Aries, is typically that everything will be accomplished immediately, and in the manner in which you expect! Over a period of time this can result in a high level of nervous strain, and it would be less mentally exhausting if you were able to slow down sometimes, and focus your energy more productively. It is to your advantage to find a calming influence in your life, maybe through the company of more placid types or some sort of activity that can provide you with the opportunity to learn patience and control. Savouring the present and directing your impetus towards the here and now, rather than seeking outer stimulus, can bring more contentment. Aries is a fire sign, and this element brings a natural vibrancy but also a tendency to impetuousness or a fiery temper. Keeping a calm head can help you to avoid clashes and misunderstandings with others, which in itself can be draining and create unnecessary tensions.

The body

Headaches are often an indication that you are taking on more than you can handle or pushing yourself too hard. In YOU CAN HEAL YOUR LIFE, Louise Hay states, 'The head represents us. It is what we show the world. It is how we are usually recognized. When something is wrong in the head area, it usually means we feel something is very wrong with "us"'. Rather than addressing any self-doubts, you might block out such feelings by driving yourself too hard. Instead of rushing into things without due thought, a relaxed attitude together with a little bit of self-understanding will result in better integration between the head (thinking and expressing) and the body (experiencing and feeling).

If you can take time out to sit still long enough, the therapy of reflexology is useful, as it can ground the excess nervous energy focused in the busy head of the typical Aries. You could also respond positively to other 'head' therapies such as cranial osteopathy or Indian head massage. Energetic sports or physical activities are a useful way of channelling and using your boundless enthusiasm, energy and competitiveness. It is of equal benefit for you to moderate

☞ *Read the Libra chapter too—your opposite sign*

your outpouring of energy with a little discrimination and keep a healthy balance between stimulation and relaxation. In general, it helps to pay more attention to your body, guarding both against accidents and against depleting your energies by rushing around in frenzied activity.

The spirit

USING YOUR INNER POWER AND FINDING YOUR SPIRITUAL MISSION

Although it is essential to release anger rather than suppress it, you can lose your inner power if you succumb easily to anger and impatience with others. Your fire and passion can be so quickly stirred that it can leave you feeling drained and miserable. Even short periods spent stilling your mind with quiet contemplation can help to build strength and patience on a deep inner level.

As you work on your soul-lesson, which is love, your inner strengths can be unselfishly employed by guiding, leading and helping others, or to a noble cause greater than yourself. By doing this, you will be furthering your spiritual and emotional growth by setting aside any selfish desires, thoughtlessness or self-centred ambitions. Until this happens, many Aries people are likely to experience lessons around love. This may be about self-loving, or learning about the correct use of love, or about how to place the needs and interests of others alongside their own. Your soul-lesson also involves being able to find correct avenues for your self-expression and the appropriate use of your power. When you are using your energies productively, your courage and tenacity and your initiating and pioneering spirit allow you to accomplish much in the world. With so much inner warmth and fervour, you have much to give others.

SUGGESTED ESSENCES
FOR ARIES SUBJECTS

Resolving possible personality imbalances

You can have a response to life so intense as to increase rather than decrease the stress in your life. You usually want things to be completed immediately, and can become impatient if they do not work out as you wish. You may be intolerant with others who perhaps take longer to understand or work more slowly than you.

Tackling impatience

Learning to understand yourself and calming and moderating your reactions can improve the quality of your life and your relationships with others.

Anger....

Waiting for anything or anyone is not easy for an Aries; you can become particularly aggravated when things do not go your way. If you are easily irritated and quick to get annoyed, **Mountain Devil** essence helps you acknowledge any angry feelings and become aware of more appropriate outlets for releasing your emotions, and in a more productive manner.

Rashness....

Black-eyed Susan essence helps you to manage your impatient energy, and reduce your tendency to a quick temper by introducing a 'more peaceful way of being'. Ian White (ABFE) makes the following comments about the type of person who would benefit from it. 'This essence can also help these people delegate work, for they have great difficulty in allowing others to take on tasks that they feel they can complete so much faster.' 'These people perceive things quickly and get irritated when those around them don't.'

Irritation....

Raspberry essence calms touchy natures that tend to react strongly to situations, especially when you are clouded by emotion. This essence replaces insensitivity with understanding and benevolence toward others.

Aggression....	Instilling a quality of maturity, the essence ***Balga Blackboy*** balances overly self-confident or forceful states. On the other hand, it encourages an individual who feels he or she needs to be more assertive. Helpful when exploring new territories or breaking into new horizons, it aids the pioneering qualities of Aries.

> *'I interpret everything that happens to me calmly and I respond with patience'.*

Calming intense emotions

Your natural spontaneity is heartening and encouraging, but your strong emotions and tendency to quick reaction can often benefit from some forethought before you respond.

Staying centred....	***Indian Pink*** essence is centering and calming to the emotions. This essence is especially helpful if you have the tendency to take on too many activities or projects simultaneously, becoming tense and stressed as a result.
Encouraging calm....	Restoring emotional balance, ***Chamomile*** essence prompts you to examine your emotions with more objectivity. Calming your fluctuating emotions, it also aids restful sleep, which can be disturbed by irritable and tense moods.
Creating composure....	***Banana*** essence encourages humility, so your judgment is not clouded by anxiety or pride. It enables an Aries to step back and observe situations calmly without becoming wound up, or responding disproportionately. This essence dissolves uptight feelings in exchange for a dignified, gentle, composed manner.
Tempering fierce behaviour....	Soothing over-emotional, competitive and aggressive states, ***Tiger Lily*** essence tempers hostile attitudes. It helps to bring peace, harmony and cooperation to argumentative states.
Instilling steadiness....	A calm, emotionally-steady nature may also be established with ***Lettuce*** essence. Not only does this essence transform agitated, excitable or angry behaviour by instilling poise and serenity, it also helps focus restless and scattered thoughts.

> *'I am serene, peaceful and centred'*

Reducing stress

Never enough time....

For people who never seem to have enough time in their lives, it is ironically the slowing-down essence **Black-Eyed Susan** that can help to create a balanced, still inner core. Its calmness enables an Aries to pace his or her energies consistently, and to cope with busy environments and situations without becoming stressed and irritated.

Unwinding....

The essence **Purple Flag Flower** is the right essence if you find it difficult to relax and release tension, especially when stressed and under outward strain. This essence helps you to control the amount of stress you can manage, enabling you to unwind and relieve excessive tension, without reacting intensely to situations.

Coping....

The essence **Hybrid Pink Fairy Orchid** helps to maintain inner peace, regardless of your outer circumstances. While preserving your sensitivity to life, it allows you to respond to situations without overreaction or emotionalism.

Relaxing....

Appropriate to speedy Aries is the Light Heart essence **Speedwell**. With this essence, harassed, rushed and agitated feelings give way to a connected sense of being in the moment. Rather than being too concerned about controlling what happens next, you may find through this essence the opportunity for you to relax your pace in life so that you are focused and concentrating on the power of the present moment.

Restoring....

The image of a **Bluebell Grove** within a wood conjures up a picture of intense blue healing energy in the mind's eye. The peace, stillness and restfulness of this space are transferred into this environmental essence, providing you with a relaxing, renewing and tranquil inner oasis. If you are in a stressed or exhausted state, then **Bluebell Grove** helps you connect with the energy of this replenishing and restorative healing space in nature.

> *'I have as much time as I need and I take everything in my stride'*

Seeing yourself in perspective

Your great enthusiasm is hugely inspiring to others, but your eagerness, together with your ambitious and self-assertive approach, usually means that you prefer to come first. Some people can find the direct, self-focused and impatient-with-limitation type of Aries difficult to deal with, as they can be perceived as superior or selfish.

Sensitivity.... **Kangaroo Paw** flower essence is for those who are so self-absorbed as to be totally unaware or insensitive of others. This essence instils kindness and sensitivity, so others sense this and feel more comfortable and relaxed in your company.

Understanding.... The flower essence **Impatiens** enhances the positive qualities of Aries. By helping you find restraint, patience and empathy, it encourages you to express your natural leadership skills with diplomacy and to manage others with understanding and tact.

Not just me.... Moving Aries subjects away from seeing themselves as foremost in life, the essence of **Spirit Faces (Banjine)** inspires a more altruistic state. It encourages the self-focused Arian to consider him- or herself with less prominence. This essence also diminishes the typical expectation of an Aries that everything should work out exactly as he or she thinks.

I am part of something bigger.... An essence that may instil a new perspective on your identity is **Lime**. Assisting you to see yourself as part of something greater than just yourself, it helps you align your skills and abilities with activities associated with collective endeavour. As your consciousness becomes more heart-based with this essence, your efforts become more focused on the needs of others.

> *'I put others first'*

Casting out self-doubt

Beneath a confident exterior there often lies a more vulnerable side, sometimes lacking in self-esteem. The lives of some

Aries people are full of never-ending activity and busy-ness. This can also be a front, hiding self-worth issues.

Self-acceptance.... Ironically, imposing and overbearing conduct is often indicative of an inferiority complex or doubting yourself in some way. In addition to its nurturing quality, **Sea Palm** essence encourages a feeling of self-acceptance and the gift of allowing things to proceed at their own pace, without trying to influence the outcome.

Self-respect.... Lack of self-esteem can also manifest in attention-seeking behaviour. In this case, **Five Corners** essence increases your self-respect and thus develops your capacity for self-love. It is helpful whenever competitive behaviour stems in fact from poor self-worth.

Self-doubt.... The positive quality that **Pineapple** essence brings is one of self-contentment, together with self-assurance and a strong sense of identity. **Pineapple** essence is perfect for the typical Aries personality, who is usually a strong character. Increasing your wise use of personal power, this essence can help you to discern your talents and strengths and the impact they have on others.

Self-empowerment.... Not only does the gem essence **Tiger's Eye** bring empowerment, it also helps you not to be overcome by your strong emotions or to react out of proportion to the emotions of others. The qualities of this essence help you keep a balance between your emotional nature and who you truly are in spirit, thus strengthening your sense of identity.

> *'I accept, respect and honour myself'*

Balancing Arian energy

A born pioneer, Aries is spontaneous, dynamic and not afraid to initiate action. Your ambition and decisiveness may make you a natural leader, and your courage and drive lead you to go where no others have dared or tried. You need to channel your energy consistently and purposefully, for otherwise you can become annoyed or discouraged, something which can be draining. In addition to finding outlets for your energy, seeking ways for inner fulfilment and taking a slower pace in life can significantly improve your vitality.

Slowing down....

Lively in nature, the Arian individual is usually considered a 'go-getter', so it is not always easy for them to appreciate the opportunities contained in the present moment.

Honouring yourself....

Cyclamen essence encourages you to be centred, and to honour your own inner needs instead of responding to the dictates of the external world. This essence offers healing if you are exhausted or burnt out from living always in the fast lane, or not nurturing yourself. It gently influences you to look at your own inner needs and to be aware of more loving and caring ways of achieving your goals.

Letting things unfold....

Impatiens essence is for slowing you down, cultivating more patience and increasing tolerance. It also lessens the typical Arian expectation that everything in life will happen promptly. It enables you to be more satisfied with just letting things in life unfold naturally.

In the moment....

A flower essence that helps reduce your tendency to impetuosity is **Verbena**. This essence draws your attention to the moment and is aptly described by Judy Griffin's affirmation which goes with it in THE HEALING FLOWERS: 'Enter my kingdom of peace'. She goes on to write that **Verbena** 'induces a meditative state .... impulsive action fades'.

Pacing energy....

Trying to do too much, you can expend your energy too rapidly and end up feeling burnt-out and frazzled. If you are the edgy, nervous, hyperactive type, or easily distracted, then *Stock* flower essence brings more fulfilment. It helps you to slow down and balance physical energy, encouraging you to pace your time and energy more efficiently.

Encouraging relaxation....

Black-Eyed Susan essence calms hyperactivity, encourages relaxation and helps you find an inner quiet place where you can reach contentment without the need for continual outer stimulus. Ian White (ABFE) links this essence with the 'Speedy

Gonzales' type, and writes the following. 'It helps people slow down, turn inwards and find the still centre within themselves, the place where they will find calmness and inner guidance.'

> *'I am content with living in the moment*
> *and letting things unfold gently'*

Providing direction and purpose

Excelling at meeting challenges and focusing on goals, you like to know where you are heading. Yet it is easy for you to become frustrated, impatient and angry when you do not have appropriate outlets for your energy or a way of channelling your power.

Which way do I go?...

With **Wild Oat** essence, you know where you are going; it puts you in touch with your purpose. It helps you to combine opportunities with talents and align them with your true mission in life.

What's next...?

Silver Princess essence guides you on your path when your direction is aimless or you are not sure of your next goal. Both *Silver Princess* and **Wild Oat** are indicated if you tend to become frustrated or despondent because you do not know where to direct and focus your energy.

Is this right for me...?

By helping you to get in touch with your true self, **Paper Birch** essence creates awareness regarding the path that is in the best interests of the person you really are. It clears outdated thoughts and conditioning, and its calming influence helps shift old belief-patterns and brings continuity of action, so you are acting for your highest good.

My purpose in the bigger plan....

Supporting your pioneering qualities, *Yellow Dryas* essence helps connects you to the bigger picture, so you can see your purpose within the larger scheme of things. It provides support so you can understand and connect your purpose to the grand plan.

> *'I know my purpose and I am guided to follow my path'*

Commitment, consistency and completion

If your attention wanes, you can become sidetracked and lose impetus for an undertaking. Ultimately, this can bring a sense of dissatisfaction, and is often exhausting when several incomplete tasks or ventures lie scattered behind you. The following essences provide dedication for the typical Aries who starts off tasks burning brightly with enthusiasm yet can fizzle out before projects are completed!

Distractions.... When you are distracted and find it difficult to complete projects, **Stock** flower essence not only enables you to expend your energies in a more balanced way, but it also assists you in bringing tasks and projects to successful completion.

Consistency.... When you are not in a position to leave the consolidation and finalizing of projects to others, or you become easily bored or distracted by new adventures, then **Peach Flowered Tea-tree** essence can help to provide consistency and the commitment to see things through.

Hyperactivity.... **Black-eyed Susan** essence (mentioned earlier) not only helps to slow down hyperactive energy, it also provides inner calm, allowing you to focus on the best way you can achieve your goals.

Fizzling out.... Perseverance and commitment to keep going is enhanced with the essence **Kapok Bush**. It brings persistence even when your energy takes a dip and you become halfhearted and apathetic.

> *'I work with consistency and I focus on completion'*

Cultivating fulfilment

Most Arians find it easier to 'do' than to 'be'. Preoccupied with the outer world and your place in it, you can find it difficult to find fulfilment and contentment on an inner level because you are not used to listening to what is truly comfortable and appropriate for you. It is to your benefit to learn the value of reflection in order to gain objectivity about life, and in handling any setbacks and delays that may come your way.

'Just being'.... **Red Huckleberry** is the essence for introspection, for withdrawing from a busy world and finding nourishment and regeneration on a deeper level. When you want to bring a new perception of what really is important, this essence promotes clear insights.

Tranquillity.... **Opium Poppy**, another red flower, correlates with the Arian energy and intensity. This poppy contains a pure white centre, suggesting an inner core of calm and peace. The essence implants this tranquil inner place into your own inner being. It helps you to assimilate past experiences in the context of your life, so that you have a greater perspective of what you have achieved and a greater understanding of how to proceed with your life. The affirmation for this essence is, 'In the midst of intense activity, I am at rest, I go forward into this day in perfect balance' (Steve Johnson, THE ESSENCE OF HEALING).

Inner contentment.... Your desire to 'do' in the outer world often overrides what is fitting for the Aries on an inner level. **Pussy Willow** essence enhances use of your intuition so you are able to synchronize your true self with your inner rhythms, and to respect what is fitting for yourself on a deep level.

Inner timing.... The qualities of **Comfrey** (LH) essence are patience and stillness. It encourages you to recognize the opportunity and beauty of each moment. It replaces feelings of impatience, eagerness or resistance with an appreciation of tranquillity and a satisfaction with the present moment. As you embrace a sense of your own inner timing, it makes it easier for you to find contentment in periods of just 'being', rather than a continual state of 'doing'.

> *'I draw in contentment and*
> *fulfilment with every breath'*

Relating and communicating

Your warmth, confidence and enthusiasm are heartening and motivating to others, but the self-centred Aries can lack consideration and support for another, which can be a stumbling-block in their relationships.

Thinking of others

The eager and passionate emotions of some Arians can mean they place their own needs before the needs of others.

Concern for others....

The essence **Fringed Lily Twiner** reduces focus on self, encouraging the demanding Arian to be less so, and to concentrate more on others. This essence instils a loving consciousness and diminishes over-concern for yourself.

Appreciation of others....

At such times as you may need to enhance your understanding and appreciation of others and their views, **Beech** essence can help. In addition to reducing arrogance, it increases tolerance towards others so that you are more able to identify with their feelings with sensitivity and compassion.

Acknowledging others....

Harvest Lily essence also provides support for the ego-motivated Arian, encouraging you to embrace another's point of view. Others will sense the even-balanced energetic influence this essence has. There is the knock-on effect of improving negotiations with others and dissolving tensions in relationships.

Consideration for others....

Promoting nurture and concern for the welfare of others, **Peach** essence increases your sensitivity and consideration. This essence instils a feeling of being secure with yourself, which in turn increases thoughtfulness and support for others. Any 'me first' attitudes or egocentricity you may have give way to concern for others with this essence.

> *'I am attuned to the needs of others
> and I appreciate how they feel'*

Cooperation with others

You like to be heard and prefer to be in charge, so enhancing your people-skills will lead to more cooperative relationships with others.

Jealousy....	Encouraging you to keep your heart open, **Holly** essence helps resolve negative traits such as jealousy, selfishness and envy by bringing patience and the ability to love without conditions.
Improving listening skills....	If you find yourself talking too much about yourself, then **Heather** essence amplifies your interest in and concern for others. The attributes of this essence encourage you to pay attention to others, be a good listener and also engage in teamwork.
Interacting with equality....	The spirited Arian has a naturally competitive side, which if it is out of balance can get in the way of relationships with others. Humility is encouraged with **Cowslip Orchid** essence, enabling Aries no longer to see things from just his or her own perspective. It also brings inner contentment, enabling the Aries to interact with others on a more equal basis, without demanding recognition from others.
Encouraging cooperation	**Tiger Lily** essence encourages you to be involved in cooperative and peaceful relationships with others, rather than displaying intolerance, which can at times be perceived as aggression.

> *'I am understanding and accommodating of others'*

Supporting and encouraging others

Consistent with your soul-lesson, placing the needs and interests of others before your own is where you can contribute best to your own inner growth. The following essences help you think of others, enhance your leadership qualities, and direct your aims and intentions to serve the positive ends of all concerned.

Increasing tolerance....	The essence **Gymea Lily** is helpful in overcoming bossiness, intolerance, dominating behaviour or the tendency to override the contributions and ideas of others. This essence increases humility, and allows you to acknowledge others but also to have your own say.
Showing compassion....	The qualities of **Peach** essence are compassion, sensitivity, concern and appreciation. It bestows interest and understanding

of others together with generosity of spirit, support and altruistic qualities.

Delegation skills....

The competitive side of your nature often means that you can end up working against others instead of with them. The essence of **Vine** helps tame those ambitious Arians who can pursue their own goals without thinking of others. Its supportive energy brings the recognition that others too must be allowed to reach their full potential. Promoting wise leadership and delegation skills, this essence encourages natural leadership and teamwork.

Positive leadership....

The qualities of self-assurance and self-acceptance that **Cowslip Orchid** essence infuses enables you to regard the successes of others as importantly as your own. This essence diminishes feelings of superiority and importance.

> *'I support and encourage others'*

Forgiving and forgetting

You put a lot of energy into most things you do, and love-relationships are no exception. It is especially important for you to feel that you are loved, yet learning to combine wisdom with love is your soul-lesson. In pursuit of this goal, you may experience some ups-and-downs in relationships at times.

Healing hurts....

If you are holding on to sorrows, then **Mauve Melaleuca** essence heals these hurts by encouraging you to be self-assured by the power of your inner self-love. This essence helps you to become more self-contained and to heal hurt feelings by replacing them with a feeling of fulfilment and contentment.

Releasing resentment....

With a little help from **Mountain Wormwood** essence you do not need to hold on to old grudges, disappointments and resentments, which can adversely affect your present relationships. This essence heals old wounds and releases bitterness.

Letting go of suspicion....

When you are overcome by feelings of revenge and suspicion, **Holly** essence tempers those emotions, softening the energy in the heart so that things can be viewed more clearly.

Resolving conflicts....

Marion Leigh refers to the keynotes of **Rowan** essence as 'Forgiveness and Reconciliation'. Addressing your attachment to emotions and patterns that do not serve your best interests, this essence helps you resolve your relationship conflicts by releasing any pain and uncomfortable feelings that accompany them.

Transforming anger....

Ian White (ABFE) writes that **Dagger Hakea** essence 'primarily brings about the open expression of feelings and forgiveness'. Particularly helpful for people who keep feelings of resentment and bitterness locked away inside themselves, this essence helps deal with anger.

> *'Any hurt feelings are dissolved and any grudges are released'*

Increasing communication skills

Dealing with defensiveness....

If you seek help in being fully present and attentive when listening and understanding to what others have to say, *Twinflower* is an ideal essence to enhance your communication skills. It is especially helpful when what others have to say may provoke an emotional or defensive reaction from you.

Communicating calmly....

Scarlet Monkey Flower essence enables you to communicate directly and calmly, without being overcome by your powerful emotions.

Easily aggravated....

Bringing detachment if you are aggravated, **Orange Spiked Pea** essence assists you to express yourself in a calm manner without uncontrollably venting bottled-up feelings, or exploding in self-defence. Know as 'the articulation of expression', 'this healing helps one to articulate feelings in a positive way and be able to walk away from a verbal fight when the only purpose from the other person is to inflict a sense of inferiority or shame. One then learns the beauty of detachment and mastery of the Self' (Barnao). Profound words for Aries subjects to ponder.

> *'I give my attention to others and communicate with objectivity and detachment'*

Authority issues

Many Arians do not like being told what to do, which may present them with problems around authority figures. Not usually needing any approval, their assertive wills enable them to act on their desires, quite often without consenting others. Finding it difficult to take orders from superiors or submit to others, they are usually ready to take the lead themselves.

Hot-headed....

Red Helmet Orchid tempers a hotheaded or selfish attitude towards those in authority. It removes your frustration and intolerance, replacing these negative qualities with consideration and respect. Together with bringing you greater awareness and sensitivity for others, it also increases and enhances your leadership qualities.

Positive expression of will....

Marion Leigh, in her description of **Rose Alba** essence, writes that 'without love, power can be misused'. She goes on to say that '**Rose Alba** is the essence of positive, outgoing, creative expression'. It assists by helping to connect you with your deep inner knowledge, in order to create a positive expression of your will. It enables you to integrate your inner power with love in order to express your truth.

Humility....

In her book, THE ESSENTIAL FLOWER ESSENCE HANDBOOK, Lila Devi calls **Banana** essence 'the humble servant'. The strong, quiet and gentle energy of this essence bestows qualities of humility and reserve where arrogance, pride or defensive characteristics exist. This essence increases your clear thinking and detachment during quarrelsome episodes, and it promotes modesty in the Arian who always needs to be right.

Diplomacy....

Instilling the right use of will in all of your actions, the essence of **Willowherb** balances an attitude of self-importance or an autocratic manner. This essence helps you to use your power with humility, diplomacy and integrity.

> *'I am humble and respectful of others'*

Resolving possible physical imbalances

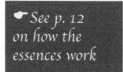 See p. 12 on how the essences work

Please note that throughout this book suggestions of a medical nature are not in any way claiming that they will cure disease, and should not be followed as a substitute to consulting a qualified medical practitioner.

Headaches

Headaches are often a signal for you that you are overloading yourself or putting yourself under stress. A constant need to rush around or achieve (typical of the Arian) can create tension, which in turn can restrict the muscles and blood-supply in the head, leading to headaches and migraines. The essence *Black-eyed Susan* helps alleviate headaches by reducing impatience and feelings of pressure. This pattern of over-exertion and strain can also be assisted by *Vervain* essence, which helps to remove the feeling of exhaustion and reduces the strain of headaches. If you cannot stop thinking about something, or for those repetitive thoughts that seem to have a life of their own, then *White Chestnut* essence quietens and clears the mind and bring relief from headaches and worry. *Mussel* essence helps relieve the irritability, frustration and anger that can also create tension headaches, and release the tightening of the jaw caused by angry feelings.

Adrenal Glands

A constant state of overactivity can stress the adrenal glands until a lack of energy results. According to Ian White (ABFE), *Macrocarpa* essence has an affinity with these glands and helps to revitalize the body. The recharging and regenerating energy of this essence not only provides energy but also brings the awareness of our need to balance activity with rest. The sea essence of *Surfgrass* supports the adrenal glands too, providing us with the courage to achieve our goals, but with a more balanced release of adrenaline. *Black-eyed Susan,* with its ability to reduce tension, has a calming and slowing-down effect that is also beneficial in adrenal stress.

Avoiding accidents

The Arian's 'busy, busy' approach can mean that it is easy for him or her to become accident-prone. It is particularly the younger Arian who is often unaware of dangers and insensitive to hazards. The relaxing influence of *Kangaroo Paw* essence helps you to develop an awareness of those times you are putting yourselves in jeopardy or taking unnecessary risks. On the same level, after taking *Impatiens* essence, you will be less bothered about rushing around and more content to take life at a reduced and therefore safer pace.

Sinus problems

Debbie Shapiro links the inflammation of sinusitis with emotional anger or irritation. She writes that 'the discharge is also emotional (fluid), a release of negative emotions or a state of being emotionally overwrought'. Eliminating such emotions helps to remove sinus problems. The essence *Eucalyptus* may ease inflammation of the nasal passages and a combination of the following Australian Bush Flower essences is suggested for sinusitis: *Bush Iris, Dagger Hakea* and *Fringed Violet.*

Blood pressure

Typically, their hot-headed emotions can mean that Arians are quick to anger, which can be a contributing factor to high blood pressure. The next two essences can help in the lowering of blood pressure: *Mountain Devil* helps release tense emotions, while *Crowea* essence brings peace, calmness and a centred feeling. *Surfgrass* essence not only brings balance and harmony to the adrenals but its properties are also supportive in helping reduce blood pressure. Dr Christine Page writes about hypertension, 'More commonly, there is an inability to be oneself for fear of not being perfect in the eyes of others'. *Five Corners,* the essence for increasing self-worth, is also suggested by Ian White (ABFH) for high blood pressure. He also advises *Mulla Mulla* essence for all 'heat' conditions.

2. THE TAURUS OUTLOOK ON LIFE AND HEALTH

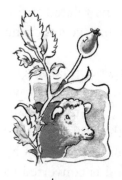

Taurus

April 20–May 21

Quality & element:
Fixed Earth

Ruler: Venus

Opposite sign:
Scorpio

Soul-lesson: Service

CONSTITUTION

ENDOWED with great tenacity and determination, Taureans can be relied on to keep going on a project or task when everyone else has given up and gone home. Their patience, endurance and persistence are their greatest strengths and ones that they employ steadfastly in everything they do. As the sign is of the fixed quality, though, they can become very stubborn in their attitudes, inflexible and set in their approach to life. This unbending nature of theirs, together with a tendency to hang on to possessions, people and situations, often originates from an uncertain stance towards life. Placing importance only in what they can see and touch, Taureans will benefit from learning to trust in their own worth and from finding security within. If they are able willingly to let go of things and people, they will find that they have all they need to sustain themselves emotionally through their own self-esteem, self-worth and self-reliance.

Implications for health

The neck, throat and ears are all ruled by Taurus, so it is important that Taureans express themselves verbally. Otherwise they can trap emotions and unspoken thoughts in these areas. Anxiety, tension or anger can often result in sore throats, laryngitis, tonsillitis, ear infections and neck problems. Debbie Shapiro, in THE BODYMIND WORKBOOK, says that throat problems have to do with an inability to speak up for what we want or to accept a reality that we do not want. Problems with the ears may also be exacerbated if Taureans do not listen to others or refuse to acknowledge or face up to what others have to say. Louise Hay (YOU CAN HEAL YOUR LIFE) writes that 'when there are problems with the neck, it usually means we are being stubborn about our own concept of a situation'. As the neck joins the head (thinking organ of the body) to the rest of the body (the doing and moving part), discomfort in this area can be related to inflexible thinking—that is, 'dis-ease' with what we are doing or moving toward.

The typical Taurean is not usually energetic, preferring a slow calm pace to life, and the comfort of his or her own home. This, along with their love of food, can render Taureans prone to weight-gain. It is essential therefore that they moderate their food-consumption, and burn up calories by keeping active, thus making sure their food is converted to physical energy. Being overweight can, at times, be due to the malfunction of the thyroid gland, and that too is linked to Taurus. This gland releases a hormone into the body that helps to regulate the size and shape of our bodies.

HEALING AND SELF-DEVELOPMENT FOR TAUREANS

The mind

If you are a Taurus, you can be acutely aware of and greatly influenced by your surroundings. This is usually the motivation to provide comfortable circumstances for yourself and those you love. Not surprisingly, with Venus—planet of beauty and harmony—influencing you, you feel happiest in a peaceful environment surrounded by rich colours and beautiful belongings. In practice, though, you may have to settle for creating this image in your mind through visualization and meditation. As Taurus is an earth sign, and therefore firmly grounded and focused on earthly survival, this is not always easy for you to achieve. If you can lift yourself out of your ordinary routine and imagine another reality, it can be a salutary experience. It can be beneficial to create a special place in your mind where you can always go to find peace, beauty and solitude. The affinity Taurus has with colour should make it easy for you to be able to use colour as a form of energy. Either in the physical sense—in clothes and belongings—or mentally, in your imagination, it can be a powerful healing tool.

It is advantageous for Taureans to put themselves into situations where they are not rushed or stressed, for this is when they operate best. They respond well to a serene and steady pace and, like all earth signs, they enjoy the calm and peace of nature. The typical Taurean relates well to the earth, so that the enjoyment of flowers and gardening as a therapy has much to offer them. For this reason, flower essences may be of special interest to Taureans.

The body

Your beauty-loving and sensual nature responds well to the physical touch, so massage and hands-on healing therapies can be ideal treatments for you. The fragrance of aromatherapy oils will no doubt appeal to the Taurean senses, so aromatherapy together with massage is an excellent therapy combination. Taurus loves to be cosseted and indulged, and a visit to a health spa or beauty farm can provide all the pampering you need to make you feel relaxed and rested. Equally, beauty therapies such as facials and manicures can boost your sense of wellbeing and make you feel special.

Taurus rules the throat, and some Taureans are blessed with a fine singing voice, which can be an excellent way of expressing themselves positively and removing tension from this area. It is equally important for non-singers to find some way in which to express themselves. For any Taurean, writing thoughts down on paper and reading them out loud can be a useful way of venting feelings and emotions and removing the tension from the throat area. Music can be most restorative, particularly if it is accompanied by some form of dance, which will provide a much-needed form of exercise. Yoga is an ideal form of exercise for Taureans, who often avoid sports and exercises that are too energetic. A creative or artistic outlet of some sort is also an important form of relaxation.

☞ Read the Scorpio chapter too—your opposite sign

Scorpio is Taurus' opposite sign, and you share some of its characteristics, including vulnerable areas of the body and potential illnesses. Like Scorpio, Taurus needs to use discrimination in sexual matters. Venus, planet of love, rules Taurus and is by its nature connected to the sexual and reproductive organs. These may therefore be vulnerable parts of the body for Taureans.

The spirit

USING YOUR INNER POWER AND FINDING YOUR SPIRITUAL MISSION

Your earthy orientation to life can mean you hang on firmly to all that you see, touch and feel, believing that it is physically lasting, safe and secure. You may cling on, desperate not to upset your sense of order and attachment to security, to such a point that circumstances may no longer make you happy and can be detrimental to your health. Your fixity of mind means that you are fearful of embracing change, and above all you need to learn trust and faith, not only of yourself but also that the universe will provide what is right for you, and when. When you learn to let go and go with the flow, you find that one door may shut but another will be opened. You can lose your inner power by missing opportunities or by blocking the chance for something better to occur in your life. Your inner power is enhanced when you can view change as a new beginning or a new opening to be embraced.

☞ For the Soul-lessons, see pp. 13 & 25

When working on your soul-lesson, your patience and practicality are excellent qualities, which can be employed in some way to provide service to others. The caring side of Taurus often enables its subjects to provide service in professions of a medical nature. Their down-to-earth, responsible and stable nature makes them reliable and trustworthy. Alongside their natural affinity with money, this is why many Taureans are often found in professions involving finance. Financial security is important to them, and it is often through money or possessions (or lack of either) that they have lessons to learn. Quite often, through some position involving money or by utilizing their own inner wealth, resources and talents they can provide a service for others.

SUGGESTED ESSENCES FOR TAUREANS

Resolving possible personality imbalances

A flexible, open mind is advantageous for you. It stops you from getting stuck in stubborn, rigid patterns, and encourages you to step more lightly through life. Increasing trust and belief in your own self-worth and your many talents encourages you to have confidence. If you are a materialistically-minded Taurean, it can be advantageous for you to seek security in other ways.

Cultivating flexibility

The Taurean down-to-earth attitude means that you can become over-conservative, even stodgy, in your thinking. It is useful for you to cultivate a flexible approach and treat everything with an open mind.

An open mind....

Wild Rhubarb essence breaks up stagnant mental patterns and allows your mind to be open to new plans, ideas and solutions. Encouraging a flow of energy between the mind and the heart, this essence relaxes your mind so that it is able to respond to deep inner guidance.

Limited thinking....

In FINDHORN FLOWER ESSENCES, Marion Leigh writes the following about **Hazel** essence. 'We often use considerable effort and energy trying to control the direction and flow of our lives, by hanging on to what has ceased to serve us, or through the limitations of our thinking.' *Hazel* essence helps you break free of limiting fears and thoughts that keep you from moving on and releasing your potential.

Over-seriousness....

Taurus is often overcautious and serious about life. This can create a rigid body as well as a rigid mind, leading possibly to arthritis or physical stiffness. An essence that helps you loosen up physically and mentally is *Little Flannel Flower*. It encourages you to perceive life with more joy and to lighten up and to trust that life can be enjoyed.

Intolerance....

Freshwater Mangrove essence also opens you to new opportunities, experiences and ideas. It frees up those Taureans that are intolerant or 'pig-headed' or prejudiced about what they believe in.

Fear....

Poison Hemlock essence helps you to move forward with a sense of empowerment, allowing you to release ingrained thought-patterns without fear, and so may be useful to Taureans.

> *'I am openminded and adaptable in my thoughts'*

Excessive concern with possessions and money

If the finances need sorting, then put a Taurean in charge; this is one of the best signs when it comes to handling money! However, when the sign is out of balance, there can be over-emphasis on the importance of money or material possessions. This often points to a lack of security or a belief that the physical and material side of life is all there is.

Balancing Materialism....

By expanding Taurean awareness, *Bush Iris* essence brings a more spiritual perspective to your thinking, which helps you maintain a healthy balance between materialism and the other aspects of life.

Security....

Also working at this level, *Trillium* essence focuses its energy on healing any obsession with the material world, by creating an awareness of spirituality. It soothes the imbalances of fear and uncertainty you may have, which can lead to a preoccupation with material possessions in an attempt to create security.

Fearing lack.... Helping to promote universal trust, belief in plenty and joy in sharing with others is the essence ***Bluebell*** (AB). This essence is for you if you feel that your reliance on physical things will ensure your survival. It works by reducing your dependence on possessions and healing any fear of lack in your life by encouraging an abundance consciousness.

Abundance.... In addition to tempering over-materialistic tendencies, the essence ***Sea Rocket*** addresses feelings of lack at either a mental, emotional of spiritual level. If your tendency is to refuse to go along with things or put up blocks, you can become stuck and unconsciously block the harmonious flow of the life-force. Losing faith in yourself or in the concept of abundance, you can cut yourself off from the flow of giving and receiving. This essence increases feelings of security and abundance, helping you to trust that the universe will provide for your needs.

> *'I have abundance on an inner level'*

Creating inner security and trust

Learning about money and possessions is part of a Taurean's life. When circumstances do not provide the sense of security he or she is looking for, it is advantageous for a Taurus to look inwards or to nature to find the sustenance that is sought.

Inner Light.... ***Windflower*** is an ideal essence for the Taurean earthly orientation to life. This essence facilitates a connection with your inner spirit, while you still keep your feet firmly on the ground, and allows you to find the light within. The affirmation for this essence, according to Sabina Pettitt's book ENERGY MEDICINE, is 'I know who I am'. It provides a sense of self-acceptance and inner security. She writes about this essence's ability 'to be in touch with heaven while being deeply connected to the earth'. Very appropriate for the earthy Taurus!

Nurture from nature.... Most Taureans enjoy gardens or relate well to nature, and this is an area where you as a Taurus can receive support and nurturing energy. *Spirea* essence works on any patterns of resistance, opening you up to the power and energy of the living world, whence you can experience nourishment and accept expansion without holding on to old methods of support. This essence is useful when you resist growth or maintain old attachments because to do so is the only way you feel supported.

Inner support....

Strengthening your inner resourcefulness, **Wild Cyclamen** essence provides for times when you have no outside support from others. It helps you to become self-sufficient and to feel nurtured. 'It encourages us to quietly seek our own counsel and to feel confident enough to trust and follow our own judgment' (Rose Titchiner, TRULY DIVINE).

Inner security....

Instilling a sense of security, **Begonia** essence supports you in letting go of possessions, by opening you up to trust in the universe and to feel less threatened by new experiences.

> *'I trust that I am looked after and supported by the universe'*

Resolving despondency or downheartedness

When things do not work out as you intend, you may become despondent and sometimes depressed. The following essences help you to tackle things at these times.

Having faith....

Gentian essence enables you to see your problems and difficulties without falling into hopelessness. It gives you confidence to see conflicts and setbacks in a different light and to realize that adverse circumstances can present challenges that, with faith in yourself, you can overcome.

Optimism....

A useful essence if you become downhearted or dejected and need lightening up is **Sunshine Wattle**. To believe that a difficult time you may have endured in the past will continue into the future creates a negative and pessimistic outlook. **Sunshine Wattle** essence allows you to perceive life differently and see the future with optimism, so that you can go forward with belief in yourself and with the faith that things will work out.

Inner joy....

The uplifting energy of **Chiming Bells** essence brings a feeling of peace and stability when you become disconnected from your inner rhythms. Its supportive strength infuses your being with inner joyful renewal if you are sad or discouraged.

Moving on....

If you feel stuck or trapped in an uncomfortable situation, you can become disheartened. Taureans are cautious people, so it can be hard for you to work out just how to make changes. **Red Grevillea** essence will provide you with the strength and courage to leave or change a situation that makes you uneasy. Ian White (ABFE) notes that the results of this essence do not always work out as one expects. 'After taking this essence, many people report that bizarre "coincidences" have occurred, which has assisted them in moving on. This is indicative of the way one's reality can change once there is a shift in one's attitudes or awareness'.

> *'Positivity and optimism pervade me'*

Boosting self-esteem and self-worth

The easily-demoralized Taurean can benefit from any boost to his or her self-worth and self-respect. The more you hold yourself in high regard, the easier it will be to have faith in your talents and the confidence to achieve more than you ever imagined.

Confidence....

Larch essence encourages confidence and clears any patterns of self-doubt or the expectation that you will fail in your future endeavours. This essence assures and empowers, so that you are no longer held back by self-limitations and restrictions. This in turn allows your true potential to blossom, and enables you to persevere when you encounter setbacks.

Expression....

An attribute of the gem essence **Lapis Lazuli** is its ability to promote clear communications in an articulate manner, thus stimulating expression if you are the shy Taurean type.

Self-belief....

Snake Vine essence creates optimism, boosts belief in yourself and reaffirms self-worth and confidence in your abilities. The encouraging qualities of this essence help you to say goodbye to self-doubt and feel positive and certain about yourself, so that you can proceed on your path without becoming demoralized or dejected.

Strength in ability....	New circumstances and changes in life are aided by *Tamarack* essence. Increasing self-identity, it strengthens your ability to carry on through challenging conditions.

> **'I am self-assured and I possess an abundance of self-esteem and confidence'**

Balancing Taurean energy

As yours is an earth sign, you operate more on the physical level. Your practical and patient outlook on life means that your energy is usually steady and enduring, but you can be resistant to change. Your calm, gentle disposition means that you do not like to be rushed; it is your nature to keep plodding on and on, often putting up with some obstacle or discomfort rather than jeopardizing your sense of security.

Breaking up sluggish and lethargic patterns

Taureans are wonderfully stoical characters, but at times they can become disheartened and weary with life, and can be notably sluggish in their feelings.

Lethargic....	Creating the feeling of being more alive and energetic, **Old Man Banksia** essence restores energy, increases enthusiasm and creates a zest for life. The following is written about those who may need this essence. 'These people have a lot of common sense. They don't rush through things, they are practical, methodical and very patient. They tend to have earthy natures and operate more from the emotional and physical planes than the mental plane.' (Ian White, ABFE). This essence thus links very well with the Taurean psyche.
Plodding on....	You can be relied upon to get the job done, but your tendency to take on more than you should means that **Oak** essence may come in useful. Refusing to give up, you may find that this work-pattern leaves you despondent and worn out. **Oak's** ability to break down fixed behavioural patterns allows you to rec-

ognize the need for flexibility instead of obstinately plodding on when it can be to your detriment.

Listless.... Changes in life can be difficult for Taurus: you may end up feeling weary and demoralized from resisting them. The essence **Stonecrop** works through feelings of resistance and attachment to how things should be, and instils stillness and patience. It enables you to cope with changes without becoming exhausted and listless.

Resignation.... If your exhaustion is prompted by a discouraged and resigned attitude, then **Kapok Bush** essence restores vitality and motivation when incentive and enthusiasm are lacking. If you feel that you cannot change a situation or tackle a problem, this essence inspires you to apply yourself to it.

> 'My vitality and enthusiasm fill me with energy'

Getting stuck

Usually Taureans are creatures of habit, with a preference for an orderly routine. This means that at times you can get into a rut and become very fixed in your attitudes and behaviour. Sometimes you become so stuck and immobile that nothing short of a rocket behind you will move you on!

Repeating experiences.... Determined in nature, you often repeat situations that you could be learning from. **Isopogon** essence helps if you are a Taurean who does not always learn from mistakes or past experiences.

Obstructions.... Stubbornly holding on to old patterns can interfere with moving on in life and can actually create blockages and stagnation in the physical body. **Jellyfish** essence encourages a fluid and adaptable attitude, allowing you to let go into an experience without putting up fixed ideas and thought-patterns as barriers and obstructions.

Unhelpful conditioning.... When thinking-patterns that are influenced by family values actually inhibit further growth and development, then **Boab** essence is instrumental in erasing any unhelpful family conditioning.

Attachments.... Washing away attachment to what has been before, the environmental essence **Glacier River** tolerates no resistance. Made from the water of an Alaskan glacier together with the fine rock particles eroded by its passage, this essence demands that Taurus goes with the flow of change. Steve Johnson says it so nicely in his affirmation for this essence: 'I willingly release that which is no longer in my highest truth. I flow with the strong, cleansing current of ever-changing life'.

> *'I put up no resistance and trust in the movement of life'*

Adapting to change

Finding acceptance of change difficult, some Taureans prefer to put up with the safety and security of what they are familiar with, even when it is uncomfortable or not in their best interests. A tendency not to trust life means they often hold on to physical things, people, beliefs and fears.

Resisting change.... **Bauhinia** essence is the appropriate essence if you resist new ideas and find it difficult to embrace change in your life. The 'hanging on' tendency may apply especially in times of alteration or transformation, when your security is threatened.

Lethargy.... When your inability to change is due more to lethargy and lack of interest, then **Kapok Bush** essence stimulates any apathetic feelings, bringing a willingness to 'give things a go'.

Letting go.... The essence of *Hyacinthus* 'White Pearl' is named **Letting Go**, and is appropriate when you need to step forward, release restrictions and limitations, and in doing so experience a positive expansion of yourself. Rose Titchiner says, '**Letting Go** helps us to realize that, like a butterfly emerging from a chrysalis, we too are on the verge of flying free into a wonderful new experience of ourselves and of the world'.

Coping with change.... Letting the past go and embracing change on any level is helped along with **Bottlebrush** essence. This essence encourages you to move on and cope with change affirmatively.

Releasing....   If you are fixed in your ways, hanging on to people and old thinking, or just finding it difficult to move on, *Lapis Lazuli* essence helps you work through these blocks by connecting you with the wisdom of your inner knowledge. This in turn creates awareness that such patterns are no longer necessary and need releasing.

Moving forward....   *Poison Hemlock* essence assists you to move forward when you have become locked into a holding pattern, particularly during periods of change, which most Taureans hate. Prompting a 'letting go', this essence is also effective in removing rigidity in your body, the build-up of excess fluids, weight and constipation.

> *'I move on, knowing that change is in my highest interest'*

Persistence and determination

Typically quiet and easy-going, Taureans usually have no lack of resolve or purpose; they just keep going and getting on with the job. After setbacks, though, they can lose their impetus and determination, and a 'what's the use?' type of apathy can set in.

Persistence....   *Kapok Bush* essence provides you with the persistence to keep going. Kicking out feelings of resignation, this essence renews the fighting spirit, so that Taurus is able to face challenges and cope with tribulations.

Endurance....   With the uplifting qualities of *Coconut* essence, endurance is increased and barriers are more easily overcome. This essence boosts energy and amplifies the motivation for completing tasks. You can 'battle on' with this essence, facing obstacles with willingness, perseverance and self-discipline.

Motivation....   When self-limiting patterns or old attachments prevent you from following through with achievements or moving ahead, then the liberating energy of *Hazel* essence can shift this resistance. In addition to instilling perseverance and motivation, it helps you to flow effortlessly along your path toward your destiny with ease. Increasing your faith to conquer obstructions, this essence inspires trust in the flow of life.

> *'I can cope with anything and have the strength of mind and the willpower to achieve much'*

Lifting up earthbound spirits

At times, it is useful for Taureans to raise their consciousness above the concerns of earthly life. So attuned are they to the physical plane that they can become bogged down and devitalized with the reality of everyday affairs and responsibilities. Allowing your spirit to fly, if only briefly, increases spiritual awareness and restores balance and inner calm.

'Living lightly on the earth....'

Marion Leigh gives the phrase 'Living lightly on the earth' as one of the messages of **Silverweed** essence. Encouraging you to live life simply, it also promotes for you a deep relationship with nature. This essence persuades you to walk on tiptoes rather than having to have two feet planted fixedly and firmly on earth. From this position, your consciousness is lifted and you can become more self-aware and grasp a vision of your higher purpose.

Feeling cut off....

If you become demoralized by setbacks, you can lose faith in yourself and become cut off from the spiritual source of abundance. When you are removed from the concept of receiving, it becomes much harder to believe in prosperity on any level. **Harebell** essence re-establishes your ability to receive and your connection to success.

A higher perspective....

The essence of **Sea Pink** shifts your consciousness away from physical concerns to trust in a higher perspective. With this essence, a more balanced energy-flow is instilled, and your ability grows to act in alignment with your highest good.

> *'I am aware of my spirituality and trust that I have everything I need'*

Relating and communicating

Characteristically quiet and not wildly outgoing, your some-what passive nature prefers others to make the running and come to you. You like your relationships and contacts with others to be peaceful and agreeable; the typical Taurean would do anything to avoid confrontation. Disputes with others can threaten his or her calm, steady disposition and sense of inner unity and tranquillity.

Maintaining harmony and peace in relationships

Harmony....
Scottish Primrose essence restores stillness when your peace is threatened in some way or if there is conflict in your relation-ship. It returns you to a state of equilibrium and inner har-mony, and replaces anxiety, shock, fear, discouragement and quarrelsome states with steady, centred energy and peace of mind.

Balance....
Lila Devi calls this 'the peacemaker'. *Pear* essence has a strong unshakeable quality, not unlike Taureans themselves. It takes a lot to stir you, but when you become troubled, disturbed and thrown off-balance, this essence reinstates poise and compo-sure. It facilitates a position of compromise, essential in resolv-ing and reconciling relationship problems.

Speaking out....
In addition to developing or enhancing listening skills, *Blue Delphinium* essence inspires courage to express yourself ver-bally, thus reducing the likelihood of imbalances in the throat. It helps you to speak with integrity and be receptive to listening to yourself.

Protection....
With a soul-lesson of service and a deep need for harmony in your life, you can benefit from the assistance of *One-Sided Wintergreen* essence. This essence not only strengthens your energy field, making you less affected by the inharmonious en-ergies of others, it also makes you more sensitive about how your own energy affects others.

'Inner harmony permeates and surrounds me at all times'

Loving without possessiveness

The Taurus subject makes a loyal and devoted partner but sometimes, in relating to others, he or she can be jealous and possessive.

Controlling....   **Chicory** essence releases controlling, demanding and overprotective attitudes, replacing them with an ability to love unconditionally and without expectation. Instilling inner security, it may enable you to feel secure enough to provide selfless devotion to the service of others, without asking for anything in return.

Jealousy....   **Mountain Devil** essence helps decrease jealousy and any attempts to cling overprotectively to others. Suspicion and frustration give way to goodwill, acceptance and kindness as this essence brings forth a consciousness of unreserved love.

Sharing....   Encouraging you in your soul-lesson of service, **Poppy (Texas)** essence assists the domineering Taurean by promoting feelings of sharing and involvement. The energy of this essence provides you with an air of positive detachment, a useful quality when you are participating in service to others.

Unhealthy patterns....   Helping you to perceive your emotions in a different light, **Yellow Pond-Lily** essence creates inner security, allowing you to release unhealthy emotional patterns or attachments. The challenge this essence helps overcome is 'attachment and doubt' and the key words are 'strength and security' (Sabina Pettitt).

Possessiveness....   An essence that encourages you in your emotional freedom, without your needing to form relationships based on fear or possessiveness, is **Bleeding Heart**. Also assisting the broken-hearted, this essence keeps the heart open and moves you toward unconditional love.

> *'I love without any expectations or demands on others'*

Shifting stubbornness

Sometimes, without being aware of it, you may use your stubbornness to control others.

Stubbornness.... *Isopogon* essence assists those Taureans who think they know best for others or when they refuse to contemplate another's viewpoint. It is also for those people who can be cast-iron in their views when they think that they are right about something. This essence releases your tendency to be bossy or controlling and facilitates flexibility and understanding in your relationships with others.

Unwillingness.... *Bauhinia* essence not only helps with resistance to change but is also useful when opposition leads to obstinate and immovable behaviour in relationships. Loosening up any reluctance and unwillingness you may feel, this essence inspires acceptance.

Uncompro- The essence of *Fig* encourages the over-serious or uncompro-
mising.... mising Taurean to become far more adaptable and openminded. The relaxing energy of this essence frees up your self-limiting patterns, transforming them with feelings of self-acceptance and comfortableness towards the self. This in turn promotes easy and flowing relationships with others.

Stuck.... Excellent at shifting attachments and detrimental patterns that can keep you stuck, resistant or stubbornly clingy in your viewpoint is the essence *Stonecrop*. It can break through these attitudes and help you release any unnecessary attachments.

Expectations.... The cooperative qualities of *Dampiera* address the belief that life and people should conform to your own expectations. The following words explain its healing abilities. 'The healing inspires the letting go of concepts that restrict the mind bringing a new quality of flexibility. Accepting and working with new attitudes becomes increasingly easier. There are then new possibilities for being deeply fulfilled and enjoying relationships with others' (Barnao). This essence promotes flexibility, and the ability to be accommodating and adaptable.

> *'I release all attachments and embrace
> all views with objectivity'*

Indulging appetites

The Taurean nature is affectionate and sensual, but when out of balance Taurus people may indulge their sensual appetites.

Balanced desires....	**Purple Magnolia** essence maintains a balanced sexual function, promoting intimacy and enhancing the senses. It is appropriate for bringing harmony to an overactive libido, but equally for those who withdraw from intimacy.
Proportion....	**Macrozamia** essence harmonizes the masculine and feminine principle in each of us, thereby creating a sense of proportion in sexual matters, in addition to helping resolve sexual inhibitions or problems such as frigidity and impotence.
Strengthens....	Whether it is habits of overeating, addictions or obsessive behaviour that you seek to address, **Blue China Orchid** essence strengthens the will. It can break old habits, helping any astrological sign—not just Taurus—create healthier patterns.
Moderation....	Sexual excesses or overindulgence in food can be alleviated by **Almond** essence. Lila Devi calls this essence 'The Self-container', because of the qualities of moderation and self-discipline it can bring. Its balancing energy instils a wholesome sexuality and behaviour that is sexually well-adjusted. She says: 'No, **Almond** does not weaken, repress or annihilate sexual energy; rather, it allows us to transmute this powerful force'.

> *'My energies are balanced and my sense of proportion is even'*

Resolving possible physical imbalances

See p. 12 on how the essences work

Please note that throughout this book suggestions of a medical nature are not in any way claiming that the essence will cure disease, and should not be followed as a substitute to consulting a qualified medical practitioner.

The thyroid

Some Taureans have a tendency to heaviness, which can be an indication of low thyroid activity. **Old Man Banksia** essence can help to rebalance and stimulate this gland and **Chiton**, a shell essence, assists when there is thyroid dysfunction. *Chiton* is also useful for when thyroid dysfunction can cause a holding pattern of excess weigh in the body. It encourages flexibility in the mind and therefore suppleness in the body.

As a gem, *Lapis Lazuli* is traditionally associated with Taurus and as a benefit in throat illnesses. Its ability to energize the thyroid makes it an excellent choice as a gem essence for Taurus.

The throat and neck

Jellyfish essence links with the throat and is an excellent essence for encouraging self-expression and communication. Beneficial for increasing creativity on any level, *Turkey Bush* essence also improves verbal expression and in doing so benefits the throat area. Other essences that work on throat problems include *Bush Fuchsia* and the gem essence *Lapis Lazuli,* both of which clear blocks in the throat area by promoting clarity of speech and bringing a conviction to speak out and express your own opinions rather than suppress them.

The essence *Mountain Devil* works to release any anger or resentment, which is important as the throat area is the Taurean vulnerable spot and grudges and powerful emotions that are held on to can stick here. Linked both with the throat and with self-expression is *Sand Dollar* essence. Assisting with positive thinking, it brings awareness of how certain belief-patterns and attitudes can go on to manifest adversely in the physical body. *Mussel* essence relaxes tense neck and shoulder muscles, while *Chiton* essence works at this level, too, breaking up blockages in the neck and shoulders and helping with neck injuries.

The ears

An essence that works physically on the ears, *Viburnum,* also increases your sense of security by enhancing your ability to listen and trust in your inner knowing.

Bush Fuchsia essence can also be used successfully to treat chronic ear infections, tinnitus and vertigo (Ian White, ABFH).

Reproductive matters

Venus, ruling planet of Taurus, rules the female sexual and reproductive organs, which can be vulnerable areas for some Taureans. *Macrozamia* essence can be used for imbalances and blockages related to these organs and their functions. Some other essences that work on reproductive problems are *She Oak, Watermelon* and *Pomegranate.*

Circulation

Venus rules the venous portion of the circulatory system, which is the deoxygenated blood that returns to the heart. Some essences that improve circulatory problems are *Five Corners, Rose Quartz, Fireweed* and *Gold.* Addressing the underlying emotional issues linked with circulatory disorders, these essences work on self-esteem (Taurus) and love (Venus). Appropriately, in THE BODYMIND WORKSHOP, Debbie Shapiro writes the following. 'As the heart is the centre of love and inner wisdom, so the blood takes that love and circulates it throughout our body; from loving ourselves we are then able to express that love and understanding throughout our world'.

Love yourself, Taurus!

3. THE GEMINI OUTLOOK ON LIFE AND HEALTH

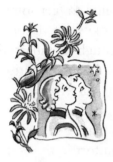

Gemini

May 21–June 21

Quality & element:
Mutable Air

Ruler: Mercury

Opposite sign:
Sagittarius

Soul-lesson:
Brotherhood

CONSTITUTION

THE LIVELY, chatty Gemini is a delightful companion, but his or her unsettled and restless side can lead to difficulty finding peace and contentment. Great talkers, Geminians have a need to communicate that often results in their tongues or thoughts running away with them, using up their vital energies. In exploring life, Geminis need variety, and will want to involve themselves in just about everything and with just about everybody, but this tendency means that they can become easily bored with the stable state. To prevent their attention and energies being dissipated, strength is called for—to establish purpose and intention in their lives. The duality associated with the sign of Gemini means that there can be two courses of action or opportunity to choose between in everyday life, a choice that Geminians may constantly debate over mentally, often finding it difficult to make a decision. This duality is also represented by the parts of the body ruled by Gemini, which are in pairs: the hands, arms, shoulders and lungs.

Implications for health

As an air sign, Gemini needs to communicate, and it is the areas and organs of their bodies associated with breathing and communicating that are most vulnerable to illness, especially when they become stressed. With their inquisitive and curious natures they exist more on the mental plane than the physical level. This causes them to live more on their nerves, so that they tend to be highly strung, sensitive or jumpy. This nervous strain may result in troubles with the lungs and the breathing apparatus. Gemini's weakness in these areas can make Gemini subjects susceptible to illnesses of the respiratory system, which may externalize as bronchitis, asthma, pneumonia, pleurisy, pneumonia or allergies. The chest area is connected with how you feel about yourself and your ability to express yourself, so difficulties in the lungs can relate literally to the inability to 'get something off your chest'. In THE BODYMIND WORKBOOK, Debbie Shapiro writes that 'when we develop a cough or inflamed bronchial tissue we are often expressing an inner frustration or irritation with how we are feeling about ourselves'.

Gemini people often use gesticulation as a form of communication, so use of the arms and hands plays a large part in their physical expression. Pain or discomfort in these appendages can be an indicator that they should be paying attention to something, while tension in the shoulder area can mean that something is a burden for them or they are shouldering more than their fair share of responsibility. In YOU CAN HEAL YOUR LIFE, Louise Hay suggests that problems with our shoulders represent our inability to carry our experiences in life joyously. Gemini people often find it difficult to commit themselves, and they need to feel free to express themselves. Feeling free to move, change and go where and whenever necessary is an essential part of their wellbeing.

HEALING AND SELF-DEVELOPMENT FOR GEMINIANS

The mind

If you are the typical Gemini, you are of a rational type. Living predominantly in your head does not always make it easy for you to be in contact with your emotions. You could benefit from visualization techniques, particularly ones involving water, which can help to involve you more with your feelings. By appreciating and paying more attention to your feelings you can bring more 'heart' into your thinking, thus creating a better balance between your emotions and your intellect.

Your mind is constantly at work on many different things at once, and therefore it does not come easy to you to slow down and focus your concentration on one thing for any length of time. To a certain extent, this is one of your lessons in life. Quietening and controlling your mind through relaxation and deep breathing can be a step in the right direction. The practice of meditation is a useful habit for you to adopt as it calms not only your mind but your nervous system also.

The body

Read the Sagittarius chapter too— your opposite sign.

A communicator at heart, you respond well to others, and among others is where you prefer to be, rather than by yourself. Therapies, exercise or sports that involve friends or a group situation are ideal for you as they give you the chance to interact with others. Generally, you would rather have fun and avoid too much discipline, so if exercise or treatment involves others, then you can be enticed in by thinking it is an opportunity to socialize. It may provide even greater appeal if you combine conversation and socializing in an environment such as a club or pub with a gentle form of exercise such as darts, snooker or pool.

Being able to communicate and express yourself freely enables a harmonious flow of energy throughout your body, which not only improves your energy levels but also creates a greater sense of wellbeing. It is useful therefore for Geminis to see conversation as a form of exercise!

Gemini rules the hands. As many Geminians are skilled at handicrafts these can provide a therapeutic occupation, as long as you can sit down long enough! Your affinity with the respiratory system positions you well for playing a musical instrument, especially one of the woodwind family. You can benefit from the breath-control that yoga offers, and from its effects of calming the mind and reducing stress.

The spirit

USING YOUR INNER POWER AND FINDING YOUR SPIRITUAL MISSION

Your busy mind is never still, constantly thinking, reasoning and analyzing. To enable you to work at your highest potential, your finely-developed powers of expression and communication need to be brought under control. Using your inner strength, you can turn off distracting internal mental chatter and listen instead to your inner voice of wisdom. If you focus with clarity on productive and positive thinking, you can rule out the internal dialogues that may be plaguing your peace of mind and contentment.

As yours is a mutable sign, you have an alert mind ready to take on new concepts, but by training your mind to be still, you can develop concentration and discrimination too. You will not then be scattering and dissipating your energies with too much talking and nervous excitement. By bringing the heart and mind together, you can become more attuned to the minds and needs of others—which helps you as you spread wisdom, through teaching, exchanging ideas or communicating harmoniously with others. In so doing, you will be working on your soul-lesson of brotherhood.

☞ For the Soul-lessons, see pp. 13 & 25

SUGGESTED ESSENCES FOR GEMINIANS

Resolving possible personality imbalances

Mercury, Gemini's ruling planet, is associated with the principles of communication, intellect and thinking. Although it makes you a quick thinker, adaptable to new situations and in taking on new concepts, Mercury's quicksilver influence can make you restless and inconsistent. Rather than be 'in your mind' all the time, you would be better advised if you learn to use the brain more as a tool or a servant. In this way you become the master, bringing it under control rather than letting it use you.

Focusing distracted minds

Often jumping from one thought or conversation to another, you can lack focus in your thinking and in your ability to give your attention to one thing or person at a time.

Distraction....

Bunchberry essence helps you become aware of how you can waste your time and easily disperse your energies when your attention is distracted, or caught up in another person's affairs. This essence restores concentration and order, allowing you to think effectively and with clarity about whatever is going on around you.

Mental overactivity....

To the typical Gemini with an overactive brain, **Yellow Boronia** essence brings a soothing influence. At the same time it focuses and centres the mind, so that you are capable of deep contemplation and reflection.

Pre-occupation....

For the mind that is agitated, scattered or preoccupied with a multitude of thoughts, **Lettuce** essence helps create inner certainty. Replacing nervousness and excitability with patience and tolerance, it helps you have thoughts that are calm, clear and concentrated. If your mind is 'all over the place', this essence teaches steadiness and tranquillity.

Focus....

When you need help to consolidate your thoughts and get to a goal, **Pink Trumpet Flower** essence can assist. It promotes clarity and purpose to realize your objectives, and it encourages inner strength. This essence has the ability to eliminate distractions from your thinking so that mental strength is consistent and the mind does not wander or lose its concentration until the job is done.

> *'My thoughts are clear, concentrated and focused'*

Balancing overly analytical thinking

Mental growth is usually important to air signs like Gemini; you need constant incentive and stimulation. In your attempt to understand life and people, or pursue some system of knowledge, your tendency is to fit everything into logical patterns. This usually stems from a feeling that nothing is real unless it can be analyzed or proven, but this narrow way of thinking can actually hold you back from utilizing your mind to its fullest potential. If you can extend your mind beyond just the mental realm, you open up to a greater awareness still.

Overly rational....

Steve Johnson advises **Lamb's Quarters** essence for when you limit understanding by perceiving things chiefly from a logical perspective. He says, 'A state of mind where the rational is over-emphasized limits an individual to one way of thinking and keeps the mental processes from being able to come into harmony with higher levels of perception'.

Narrow thinking....

All knowledge serves us best when combined with emotional experience, providing inner wisdom and truth, rather than the acquisition of facts from a plausible basis only. Creating this desirable balance between the mind and the heart, **Hibbertia** essence integrates intuition with ideas and rationality, enabling you to become more flexible and less narrow in your thinking.

Integrated thinking....

Mercurial people, Geminians are often involved in intellectual professions such as writing or teaching. The quality of **Shasta Daisy** essence helps the mind incorporate separate areas of knowledge and information perceived from a purely analytical perspective into a more complete and integrated whole. Assisting Geminians in their mental work, it helps an overall picture emerge rather than scattered pieces of information and isolated facts.

> *'My awareness opens me to higher levels of perception'*

Destroying vacillation and indecision

It is in your nature to have two, if not more, things on the go at the same time. Often dithering between two decisions or options, you can be indecisive and ambivalent.

Focus....

Helping you judge whether a certain course of action is the right one to take, the essence *Jacaranda* brings a quality of focus. Its centering ability aids you in making decisions without excessive wavering or continual consultation of others, and helps you stick with one decision rather than repeatedly changing your mind.

Concentration....

The flower essence *Lettuce* not only brings you patience, concentration and decisiveness, it also enhances Gemini's communicative abilities by ensuring you express yourself in a clear, sure manner.

Consistency....

With so many options and choices in your life, you can benefit from the decisive qualities of *Scleranthus*. This essence, which restores a sense of inner balance, not only helps you to act decisively and reliably, but also calms changeable, restless and unfocused energy. For the Geminian who is unreliable—maybe chopping and changing their moods, opinions or subjects of conversation—this essence encourages consistency and calm inner direction.

Decisiveness....

A lovely affirmation for the essence *Pipsissewa*, taken from ENERGY MEDICINE by Sabina Pettitt, is this: 'I am able to choose. I can trust my energy and follow my heart'. The decisive energy in this essence dissolves the anxiety around decision-making, helping you to make the right choice. Sometimes, in taking a decision, you may be unable to see the bigger picture and things do not always turn out as you think they should. In these circumstances, the wisdom of *Pipsissewa* helps you move from dissatisfied and confused states to knowledge about which move to make next.

> *'I know what to do and I stand firm in my decisions'*

Having a tendency to live predominately in your head, you can become separated from your feelings and isolated from your emotions.

Blocked emotions....

According to Ian White (ABFE), people needing **Yellow Cowslip Orchid** 'are focused so much in their intellect that they are often blocked off from many of their feelings'. This essence opens the Gemini mind with humanitarian concern for others; it is also useful in freeing up critical and judgmental natures.

Too focused in the head....

In the same book, Ian White says the following about those people needing the essence **Hibbertia**. 'the energy of these people is focused in their heads more than in any other part of their bodies, especially their hearts'. He goes on to say that '**Hibbertia**e helps to drain excess energy from the mental plane in order to balance the emotional plane'.

Balanced feelings....

The ability of **Bush Fuchsia** essence to integrate the left and right hemispheres of the brain is helpful to the Geminian, who may function mainly from a logical, rational perspective (left side). When there is a better balance with the intuitive, creative side (right side), you can trust gut feelings and express yourself with more insight from your intuition.

> *'My heart is open and I am connected to my feelings and emotions'*

Your affinity is with the mind, which ceaselessly moves from one thing to another. Your need for mental stimulation finds you most comfortable in the world of ideas and abstract thoughts. It is your constant inquisitiveness and curiosity that prompt your talkative and restless nature, often leaving you no time to find trust in your own truth and wisdom.

Inner certainty....	Your distrust in your own judgment means that you often need confirmation from others when making decisions. *Cerato* essence brings certainty and concentration to the Gemini mind, so you will be able to believe in your own inner guidance, rather than striving to find assurance from others. This essence helps your inner sense grow, allowing you to get in touch with your own intuition and impressions. These insights, combined with your rational mind, allow you to make the right decision or do the right thing.
Trust....	Strengthening the connection with your inner voice, **Viburnum** essence increases intuition and heightens awareness so you will be able to stop, listen and trust in your own inner voice. Another advantage of this essence is that it calms the nervous system—which in Gemini's case can easily become tense, jumpy and 'frazzled'.
Clarity....	The sea essence *"Staghorn" Algae* brings the ability to perceive a sense of yourself from a higher perspective, particularly when you are surrounded by confusion or in the midst of mental turmoil. It also promotes clarity in your thinking and improves decision-making.
Intuition....	Finding your source of wisdom within is aided by *Scots Pine* essence, which opens clear channels to inner listening. This essence enhances your intuitive powers and increases your inner certainty. Lessening your reliance on outside validation, it increases receptiveness so you are guided to listen to inner truths.

> *'I trust in my inner guidance and I am
> guided by my intuition'*

Balancing Gemini energy

Gemini's wonderfully expansive mind is a versatile and enquiring one. Preferring variety to routine, you love change and can easily find yourself diverted in some direction of thought other than the one you intended. Although Geminians are not usually lovers of regimentation, being able to control your mind is advantageous, otherwise you can end up scattering your forces and draining your energies.

Battling with bored and restless natures

You are eager to experience as much as you can, and your flexibility enables you to adapt effortlessly to new situations, while your variable nature can easily make you bored. If you undertake too many new commitments or tasks you can dissipate your resources and become unproductive.

Lack of purpose....

If you are dissipating your energies through unclear purpose, the antidote for this sort of behaviour is **Jacaranda** essence. This is the correct essence for the Gemini who ends up with several incomplete projects rather than mastering one thing well. The positive quality of poise this essence instils assists you to take on only those actions that you can complete successfully. Rather than rushing around madly, yet not actually accomplishing anything, you can maintain a clear head and focus on achieving.

Unpredictable nature....

Peach-Flowered Tea Tree essence replaces the Gemini tendency to unpredictability and to fluctuation from one extreme to another. It instils continuity where inconsistency and boredom exist, making it easier for you to follow projects through rather than lose interest and waste energy.

Lack of discipline....

In order for you to be able to complete undertakings without getting frustrated and giving up easily, the assistance of **Wandering Jew** essence produces the necessary discipline and patience. It enables you to be able to combine your ideas and reasoned thinking with consistent energy, facilitating you in all your endeavours and leading to achievement.

Poor reliability....

Replacing restlessness and disinterest with persistence and willpower, the essence **Kapok Bush** provides the effort, strength of mind and resolve to stick with something if you tend to be unreliable, apathetic or disinterested.

> *'I have self-discipline and I use my energy with consistency and wisdom'*

Settling mental gymnastics

A busy head, full of churning thoughts, not only depletes Gemini's life-force but can make sleeping difficult and disturbed.

Mental exhaustion....

Nasturtium essence restores vitality when you find that continual mental hyperactivity and gymnastics exhaust you.

Persistent thoughts....

Quietening the mind, **Boronia** essence releases persistent unwanted thoughts and replaces them with peace and stillness, which support restful sleep. It brings clarity, helping you clear your mind of obsessive thoughts and enabling you to tune into your intuition more.

Internal chatter....

Promoting a quiet, calm mind, **White Chestnut** essence turns off the internal chatterbox, allowing you to let go of constant, useless gnawing thoughts and replace them with tranquillity and clarity. This essence eases the tendency to go over the same problem again and again, or continual thinking about what you might or should have said or done in a certain circumstance.

Quiet mind....

It is difficult for many Geminis to stay quietly in the moment without thoughts of what is likely to happen next. The environmental essence **Polar Ice** brings about a quality of stillness where you are unattached to anything beyond the present moment. This reflects the environment and conditions near the North Pole, where this essence was made: completely remote without distractions, invoking feelings of 'time just standing still'.

> *'I am calm, peaceful and focused only in the moment'*

Calming erratic nervous energy

It is typical of a Gemini to be involved in trying to do too many things at once, resulting in spurts of unpredictable energy that can adversely affect their consistency and stamina. In the extreme, this predisposition can drain the nervous system and can result in mental or physical collapse. It is important that you sustain a constant state of energy output to keep up with your many activities.

Taking time.... Appropriately named if you are the overactive Gemini, rushing around, *Speedwell* essence teaches you to 'take your time'. Rose Titchiner writes, '*Speedwell* can profoundly change our experience of time. When we let go our feeling that there isn't enough time, extraordinary things happen in the shortest enriched moments of being'. This essence helps you connect with the present moment, and enables you to have 'the time of your life' without tension, stress or the limitation of time.

Stable energy.... Matching vitality with consistency, *Purple Enamel Orchid* essence introduces a stable output of energy, ensuring concentration and steady progress towards achievement. This essence sustains vitality and stamina by regulating the appropriate balance between work and rest.

A healthy pace.... The advantage of *Hops Bush* essence is that it can re-establish a healthy pace to your energy system, without overstimulating your mind. It enables you to feel calm and peaceful, yet have sufficient balanced energy to complete your various interests.

Moderation.... Helping Gemini focus on one thing at a time, *Almond* is the essence for self-control and moderation. Aiding you in wise use of your time and energy, this essence helps produce an output of energy that is calm and relaxed.

> 'My pace is gentle and steady and
> I take one thing at a time'

Inducing a meditative state

It is to your advantage, if you can manage it, to be still and present in the moment, if only for a short period at a time. Concentrating on observing your breath and focusing your thoughts away from everyday cares and activity is immensely helpful when you can make a regular practice of it.

Serenity.... The gem essence *Aquamarine* can assist you in achieving a peaceful meditative state. Incorporated into your daily routine, such meditation can have huge benefits. Reaching a point of calm where serenity and stillness flourish, the essence creates a clear receptive mind free of repetitive thoughts and overstimulation.

Turning inwards....	**Cassandra** essence encourages stillness of the mind, brings deep relaxation and the ability to receive inner guidance in meditation. It enables you to turn your mind inwards so you can gain new insights, move beyond your usual perceptions and attune more deeply with nature.
Receptivity....	Helping to integrate the conscious mind with the unconscious mind, **Lady's Mantle** essence can expand your awareness. This essence encourages you to be receptive to your inner world of feeling and helps you open to a spiritual perspective, thus increasing your ability to contemplate and reflect. It provides you with a better understanding of your true self on a deep level.
Tranquillity....	The image of a **Bluebell Grove** conjures up a picture of intense blue healing energy. The stillness and restfulness of such a space are transmitted by this environmental essence, providing a relaxing, renewing and tranquil inner oasis. If you are in a stressed or exhausted state, this essence helps you to connect with the energy of this restorative healing space in nature.

> **'I can create a state of tranquillity
> and peace whenever I wish'**

Lighthearted living

Life's complexities and problems may dampen your spirit and weigh down your energy. If you are a typical Gemini, you like to be carefree and lighthearted, as this state is the one in which you operate best.

Playfulness....	**Zinnia's** uplifting qualities restore humour and laughter and a childlike playfulness at heart. It recaptures lightheartedness if you become over-serious and heavy.
Joy....	Connecting with your inner child, **Little Flannel Flower's** carefree qualities restore playfulness and joyfulness. With attributes of spontaneity and cheerfulness, this essence helps you to express elation and increased enjoyment in life.
Looking on the good side....	The ability to see life from a perspective of fun and goodwill, even in difficult and stressful situations, can be restored by **Yellow Flag Flower** essence. Helping you to find humour or to look on the good side of things, this essence assists you to

GEMINI (MAY 21–JUNE 21) · 81

remain strong, cheerful and untroubled despite everyday pressures or worries.

Uplifting.... The name of the essence **Fairy Bell** conjures up lightness and flitting, dancing energy, and the key phrase for this essence, according to Sabina Pettitt, is 'Lightness of Being'. Ideal for Gemini, the energy of this essence not only lifts a feeling of heaviness, it also frees the lungs and eases the breathing.

> *'I am happy-go-lucky and cheerful and dance lightly through life'*

Relating and communicating

With your innate ability to communicate and spread the word, you may realize that Gemini plays an important part in our spiritually-evolving world. In this regard, respect for others is vital and an appreciation of their needs is fundamental in your communications with them.

Your networking mission is to convey spiritual insights and wisdom to others. Before you can do so, you need to move into a position of clarity and to be able to transmit knowledge from the highest and most profound source.

Instilling wisdom and clarity in your communications

When working on your soul-lesson of brotherhood, you need to be able to impart your knowledge to others clearly, with compassion and wisdom.

Listening.... **Twin Flower** essence helps you to listen effectively and to clarify your thoughts. The positive qualities of this essence can inspire you to communicate with others from a position of inner refinement and calmness.

The wisdom in silence.... Others often have trouble keeping up with fast-talking Geminians, who may need to learn the wisdom of silence and to quieten their tongues on occasions! The calmness that **Lettuce** essence brings allows for a better balance in interpersonal relationships as it allows impatience to give way to patience and tolerance for others—quieter yet able to express your truth clearly.

Expressing suppressed thoughts....

Blue Delphinium essence inspires you to speak out with honesty, integrity and sincerity. It conquers the fear of speaking your truth and it enhances the ability to listen effectively to others and to yourself. Thus it becomes easier for you to know just how and when to respond and when to remain silent. It helps you voice suppressed thoughts and remove inhibitions associated with speaking, singing, writing or listening.

Co-ordinated thoughts....

Sorting out the host of ideas, thoughts and intentions that you can carry in your head, the essence **Broom** tackles this tangle by encouraging coordination and integration of thoughts. '**Broom** essence stimulates mental clarity and concentration, facilitating ease in communication and creative thought when in a state of bewilderment' (Marion Leigh). This essence helps decision-making, enhances creative thought and enables intuition to illuminate your mind. It thus promote clear purpose and guidance.

Articulated speech....

A powerful essence for communication, **Cosmos** is the ideal essence for the fast-talking Gemini. Your mind moves so quickly that you can have trouble verbalizing everything you want to say coherently. **Cosmos** essence assists you in organizing efficiently and integrating disorganized thought-patterns into articulate speech.

> '*I listen with patience and communicate with wisdom*'

Communicating with heart energy

When listening to and understanding others, subjects of air signs like Gemini work from a rational point of view, which can tempt them to shy away from their emotions.

Connecting with others....

Tall Yellow Top essence is significant for this sense of alienation, as it reconnects the head with the heart. Helping you unite with others more easily, this essence permits you to communicate from a balanced position of mind and heart energy.

and with the feelings....

Flannel Flower's positive qualities enable you to express open, sensitive and gentle feelings in your physical and emotion interactions with others. Enhancing the ability to share your feelings, it is for people who do not feel comfortable with them and may draw away from physical closeness.

Releasing emotions....

If you are sad or grieving, it can constrict your vulnerable chest area and inhibit your ability to express your emotions articulately. *Yerba Santa* essence alleviates these bottled-up and stifled feelings, allowing the heart to feel lighter and your emotions to flow more freely.

Being comfortable with the intuition....

When thoughts are detached from feelings, the flower essence *Mallow* unites the mind with the intuition, enabling thinking to be guided from the heart. This essence also addresses repetitive thoughts and being 'too much in the head'.

> *'My thoughts and heart are aligned and I am comfortable with my feelings and emotions'*

Straight talking

In mythology, Gemini's ruler Mercury is the speedy messenger of the gods, so no wonder Gemini people are fast movers and fast-talking conversationalists! Never at a loss for words, 'smooth-talking Mercury' can also be crafty and devious with his or her words at times. A wily mover with a glib tongue, the mercurial type can resort to gossip, fickleness or being elusive with the truth, substituting his or her own words to suit personal needs.

Honesty....

The key words for *Easter Lily* essence, according to Sabina Pettitt, are 'truth, purity, integrity and honesty'. This essence is about expressing your true being, without having to play a role, put on a mask or use duplicity in your words. If you are one of those Geminis who can be superficial, flippant sometimes, this essence inspires you to respect in your dealings with others.

Straight-forward talk....

Instilling a sense of honesty, *Fuchsia Grevillea* essence ensures that interactions with others are straightforward and truthful. This essence helps create for you a complete unity between thoughts, words and deeds, as aptly described by the meditation poem for this essence. 'As I think so I become. | To fill the mind with loving thoughts | brings loving words | brings loving deeds | in such a world I want to live' (Barnao).

Goodwill....

If Gemini's curiosity gets the better of you, resulting in unhealthy gossip and interference in the affairs of others, then *Fringed Mantis Orchid* essence awakens the conscience. It restores goodwill and kindness, so your mind works only with the best intentions towards others.

> *'I communicate always with honesty and integrity'*

Creating consistency

A typical Gemini has a continual need for interaction with many different people. This, together with their restless search for direction through others, is why they can often be seen as inconsistent and unreliable.

Accountability....

The settling qualities of *Christmas Tree–Kanya* essence can inspire you to fulfill your responsibilities consistently. This essence produces a feeling of contentment with being accountable, and its reliable, caring energy ensures that any selfishness gives way to sharing and concern for the needs of others.

Dependability....

Strawberry essence has a centring ability, which brings inner strength and self-acceptance, resulting in behaviour which is dependable and committed. This essence replaces uncentred, indecisive or irresponsible conduct with decision, sureness and steadfastness.

Self-reliance....

Helping to implant self-reliance and self-approval, *Illawarra Flame Tree* essence encourages responsibility and commitment to a course of action. It enhances your sense of inner strength, so you are able to cope with issues in life without opting out because of the responsibility involved.

Constancy....

Marion Leigh refers to the essence of *Laurel* as having a harmonizing and synthesizing effect. The energy of this essence enables you to put your ideas into action without being distracted and giving up. It instils strength, commitment and constancy.

Handling commitment

A typical Gemini is unemotional and therefore can be rather noncommittal about attachments to others. Instead of you pulling away or becoming overwhelmed when dealing with relationships, your strength and dedication are called for. Preferably, Gemini needs a partner who respects their need for freedom, variety and self-expression. Within this framework, these essences can assist those Geminis who wish to promise their allegiance or pledge their loyalty.

Commitment....
: **Many-Headed Dryandra** essence focuses on bringing together your fulfilment with the consistent commitment needed in longterm relationships. Especially suitable if you tend to run away from facing responsibilities in relationships, this essence encourages dedication and stability.

Dedication....
: The aptly-named **Wedding Bush** is the essence if you are one of those Geminians who have trouble committing in relationships, or if your inconsistency actually sabotages the satisfaction you seek in relationships. This essence is helpful either in binding attachments within your existing relationship or in helping you to stop going from one relationship to another. It is also useful in bringing dedication to a goal or life-purpose.

Devotion....
: Deepening your connections with others, **Pearly Everlasting** is the essence to instil devotion and fidelity. Sabina Pettit writes, 'this remedy can be especially helpful to those who feel unwilling and/or unable to make a deep and lasting commitment in relationship'.

Procrastination....
: **Coconut** essence is the answer to lack of commitment, finding excuses or an escapist attitude. It deals with procrastination and provides patience, endurance and willing realism. This essence replaces a noncommittal attitude with a sense of readiness to deal with issues and honour commitments and vows.

Resolving possible physical imbalances

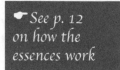*See p. 12 on how the essences work*

Please note that throughout this book suggestions of a medical nature are not in any way claiming that the essences will cure disease, and should not be followed as a substitute to consulting a qualified medical practitioner.

The nervous system

If you are a Gemini with a highly-strung, nervy disposition, you can benefit from the composing qualities of **Morning Glory** essence. Calming the nervous system, this essence replaces restlessness and agitation with ordered calm. It brings a sense of stability to daily routines and it regulates good sleeping habits, especially for those Geminis that tend to burn the candle at both ends. The calming qualities of **Chamomile** essence help to alleviate stress in the nervous system and to create emotional harmony. In addition to reducing tension, this has the knock-on effect of strengthening the vulnerable respiratory area.

Iris essence aids in releasing mental seriousness, bringing a more balanced approach mentally and physically. Working to stabilize the nervous system, **Coffee** essence not only nullifies caffeine in the physical body (which can interfere with the effectiveness of flower essences) but it also reduces dependence on caffeine.

The quality of **Almond** essence is one of moderation and balance and can assist those who spread themselves too thinly, resulting in nervous tension. **Boronia** essence releases unwanted, persistent thoughts with peace, stillness and restful sleep.

The arms and shoulders

The Gemini personality who needs a logical or analytical explanation for everything is often prone to mental strain. This leads to stress and tension in the shoulders and arms.

Dampiera essence releases tight muscles, cramps and spasms, and reduces pain in these areas. This essence can be used topically and is a constituent of *The Australian Living 'Body Soothe' Cream* (AL), which is invaluable for aches and pains. The sea essence *"Staghorn" Algae* not only helps produce clear thinking, it also works physically to relieve tight and painful shoulders.

The respiratory system

Air signs need plenty of oxygen and are usually the ones flinging open the windows in order to get the air circulating in a room! The essence *Sturt Desert Pea* can be used for breathing difficulties as it allows sadness, grief and loss to be released. All of them feelings can adversely affect lung function. By facilitating a healthy expression of our emotions, this essence frees up even those feelings that have been suppressed for a length of time. *Yerba Santa* essence helps repressed emotions flow more easily, and this can have the effect of lightening your demeanour and shifting chest congestion, even pneumonia, at the same time.

Green Rose relieves the fear which can often impact one's breathing resulting in respiratory problems, while *Babies' Breath* brings energy to the lungs, helping with conditions such as asthma, bronchitis or pleurisy. Bronchial conditions can also benefit from the assistance of *Polyanthus*, *Sand Dollar* or *Tall Mulla Mulla*. With its ability to propel mucus and inhaled particles out of the respiratory system, *Carrot* essence works on enhancing the efficiency of the respiratory passages. *Spike Lavender* essence concentrates on clearing lung congestion and *Tansy* essence works on conditions such as emphysema.

The thymus

Gemini is linked with the thymus gland, which sits in the chest cavity, close to the heart, and is involved in the body's immune response. It is responsible for fighting bacteria, viruses and other germs. Sabina Pettitt mentions *Jellyfish* essence as one that acts on the thymus to balance the immune system, in her book ENERGY MEDICINE, while *Illawarra Flame Tree* essence strengthens this gland also.

4. THE CANCER OUTLOOK ON LIFE AND HEALTH

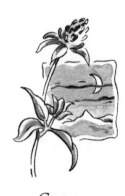

Cancer

June 22–July 23

Quality & element: Cardinal Water

Ruler: the Moon

Opposite sign: Capricorn

Soul-lesson: Peace

CONSTITUTION

CONCERNED, kind and protective, Cancerians often instinctively know what another person needs, and excel at administering and caring for others. Intuitively, they know exactly when to reach out to those who need help, yet at other times they can withdraw completely into their own shell. As Cancer is a water sign, feelings and emotions are uppermost in their approach to life. This, together with their sensitive and sympathetic manner, makes them very receptive to others' thoughts and views. They can be so vulnerable that they can easily absorb the concerns and worries of those closest to them. It can be very easy for them to take everything to heart, so that they sometimes respond moodily or defensively, and take things more personally than was meant. Since Cancer is categorized as a cardinal sign (see p. 25), Cancerians often have enterprising spirits and will usually be ready to instigate and move forward in life, but the fearful Cancer can worry unnecessarily about anything and everything. It is important that they learn to overcome any fears, as anxiety can drag them down emotionally and physically.

Implications for health

Cancerians' tendency to worry can cause them digestive problems, indigestion and ulcers, sometimes even eating disorders. It is crucial that they express their emotions in order that any fears and tensions are released, instead of their being absorbed into their bodies. Cancer rules the chest area, stomach, digestion and those parts of the body that involve nourishment or nurturing of the self or of another (e.g., the womb and the breasts, as they are used in breast feeding).

Cancer's affinity with family can put its subjects in positions in which they become deeply involved with family members, be those members children, elderly parents or siblings. Whatever the family issue, Cancer often shoulders more than its fair share of the responsibility. Yet Cancerians may take it in their stride, and they are usually more than happy to be entrusted with such responsibility—to the extent that many Cancerians are to be found in professions that involve nurturing and the care of others in some way. Balance is essential here, though, as they often derive their own emotional satisfaction from being needed. They therefore have to learn exactly how much to give others and how much to save for themselves, if they are not to become totally exhausted and drained with the demands of others. Fulfilment, wellbeing and inner emotional contentment are achieved by reaching a point of calmness in their emotions and in employing their qualities of nurturing and caring for others in a balanced manner. Their sensitivity to others means that being in the company of positive people is important. It is beneficial and uplifting for them to be with optimistic people, as Cancer will naturally absorb their favourable moods.

HEALING AND SELF-DEVELOPMENT FOR CANCERIANS

The mind

If you are a typical Cancerian, then you are very open to the feelings, actions and thoughts or others. It is crucial that you have your own sanctuary—either physically or mentally—

where you can get away from all those who so easily deplete your energies. Your extreme sensitivity and awareness can be wearing, to the point that you become easily devitalized by worry and fear. It is helpful for water signs like Cancer to work constantly on visualizing a protective field of golden light around themselves, which guards them from being drained by the invasive energies of others.

As a Cancer, you may live in a world that is coloured by a glorified past. A world that was either so marvellous that it never matches up to your current life or so awful that you drag it behind you like a ball and chain. In accepting that the past has gone, you can direct positive thoughts into shaping your future; it also helps to know what you actually want. If you find it impossible not to worry, then practise striking out mentally each negative thought as it arises, and correcting your thoughts affirmatively. It is useful for you to use your imagination constructively by practising affirmations (like those in this book), which are repetitive, positive declarations that purposefully focus and programme your mind. This can only help, as you will be influencing the future by investing positive thought and energy into it.

The body

Water signs (Cancer, Pisces and Scorpio) often seem to be drawn to spending time in or close to the ocean or some body of water. This element is healing, so all pursuits involving water can help you to release physical and emotional tensions. Therapy pools may appeal; hydrotherapy pools to stimulate the circulation and thalassotherapy pools (which include a salt-water jet massage) can ease pains and restore and energize tired bodies. Swimming can be strengthening, especially to the chest area, often a vulnerable area for Cancer. Not surprisingly, the chest is associated with our sense of identity, so it is important that Cancerians learn to create a strong sense of self.

Most Cancerians love to cook, but they may tend to use

☞ Read the Capricorn chapter too— your opposite sign.

food for emotional security. Eating when agitated and nervous is likely to result in digestive problems and upset stomachs, so should be avoided. Water signs in general can be prone to poor elimination and Cancer is no exception. This can have a lot to do with the inability to release old emotional patterns and the readiness to let go of the cords that keep one bound to the past. Regular exercise can help to eliminate excess fluids and the breakdown of fatty tissue.

Cancerian carers themselves respond well to the loving attention of others, and particularly through an experience where physical 'hands-on healing' is used. Looking after another person, animal or plant is itself a salutary experience for the Cancer person, who loves to have someone or something to nurture.

The spirit

USING YOUR INNER POWER AND FINDING YOUR SPIRITUAL MISSION

☞ For the Soul-lessons, see pp. 13 & 25

If you have a tendency to dwell on the past, or worry or fantasize aimlessly over the future, then you could be wasting your inner power. If you are going to embrace your soul-lesson of attaining inner peace, you need to release old attachments and step into the reality of the here and now.

Being tossed perpetually around like a boat in a high sea of emotions, Cancerians can feel that they are at the mercy of their feelings. If you are Cancer, then like the subjects of other water signs, your quest is to attain some sort of inner peace from these turbulent emotions. This will quite likely be your life's journey, as you learn the best way to overcome and handle your vivid imagination, self-inflicted worry or the invading energies of other people.

Most important, as a nurturer of others, you need to appreciate and nurture yourself first. You need to provide yourself with a sense of peace, calm and inner strength and security before you extend your calling to nurturing others.

SUGGESTED ESSENCES FOR CANCERIANS

Resolving possible personality imbalances

Greatly influenced by your vivid imagination, you often believe the worst will occur. Living in your emotions, and with your innate sensitivity to everything going on around you, you can easily become consumed with anxiety, dread and fear. To handle this outlook on life you need to utilize good calming techniques—and employ large doses of rationality—to ensure that your fears and worries do not overwhelm or debilitate you.

Banishing worry, anxiety and fear

Easily troubled or distressed, the irrational Cancerian could win a gold medal for worry!

Anxiety....

The relaxing essence **Crowea** is ideal for coping with troubled or anxious states and the perfect choice in helping to restore us to a calm centre. In the persistent worrier, it allays irrational thoughts and instils emotional balance and peace.

Nervousness....

Succumbing to the workings of your wild imagination, your thoughts and your perceptions, you can become fearful of just about anything. Vague fears can seem to arise from nowhere; this uneasiness can make you apprehensive and fearful about life in general. **Aspen** essence dispels feelings of nervousness and unease, enabling you to feel secure enough to tackle life without fear. It brings a sense of security and enables you to trust that you are safe and protected—just how Cancer prefers to feel.

Fear....

The essence **Bog Rosemary** instils deep trust that you are safe and protected. It provides support if you become immobilized by irrational fears of the unknown. It enables you to take risks and move through life with faith, in order to grow or to heal.

Trepidation....

The comforting quality of **Red Clover** essence brings awareness of just how fear excludes one from experiencing what is good in life. '**Red Clover** shows us just how powerful our thoughts are, and how our thinking affects our experience and the energy that we resonate to the world' (Rose Titchiner). If you are in trepidation—in dread of or overwhelmed by events around you—the message of this essence is 'all is well'. It helps you to perceive events with positivity rather than fear.

> *'I have nothing to fear and I trust that I am safe'*

Calming emotions and developing detachment

The nature of the Moon, Cancer's ruler, is that of change and fluctuation. This can be seen through its effect on the tides, ebbing and flowing, advancing and retreating. Cancer's moods vary also; you can be elated one moment and flattened the next. Learning to calm overwrought emotions and obtain a degree of detachment is vital to your ability to cope with life harmoniously.

Stability....

Chamomile essence creates stability. It renders you capable of handling these changeable moods, or emotional extremes. It increases your emotional objectivity, decreases moodiness and infuses you with a sense of inner peace.

Soothing....

With a most fitting name for Cancer, **Moonstone** is a potent gem essence for working with anxious emotions. Lessening identification with the emotional state, this essence brings a degree of control over your emotions. Its balancing and soothing properties also help to bring suppressed emotions safely to the surface, to be resolved rather than unconsciously expressed.

Composure....

A calm, tranquil, emotionally steady nature may be achieved with **Lettuce** essence. Not only does this essence transform agitated, nervous, excitable or troubled emotions by instilling composure and serenity, it helps focus restless and scattered thoughts. *Lettuce* essence aids you in learning to control your thought-processes, rather than letting them run wild. '**Lettuce** also offers the antidote to an indecisive mind; inner certainty. Remove the anxiety, fear, and attachment to the outcome of a decision, and you have an individual with all the knowledge— or the ability to gather it—needed to resolve most any problem' (Lila Devi).

> *'My emotions are balanced and I feel calm and peaceful'*

Cutting through the fog

You experience life mainly through your emotions. Responding to sensations, you tend to feel and intuit rather than think on a purely logical basis. Your extreme sensitivity and vulnerable emotions can often lead you to withdraw when you encounter the harsh realities of life.

In a dream.... **Sundew** essence helps you stay focused in the real world, instead of living mentally absent from it, caught up in some vision, dream or impression. This is not to say that your imagination is not important. This essence can be beneficial in learning how to channel this form of inspiration consciously and to bring these thoughts into practical reality.

Fantasy world.... You can be elsewhere in your thoughts, dreamy, living in your own world, somewhere in the past or in some idealized future in your imagination. The flower essence **Clematis** addresses inattention, indifference and confused states, helping to bring the unrealistic or idealistic Cancer back into reality. It helps you to utilize your colourful imagination realistically and to be able to ground your vision and make it workable. This essence enables you to live more in the present and easily handle any unpleasant situations that may arise, without escaping to some fantasy world.

Inattention.... **Avocado** (SN) essence helps the faraway or spacey Cancer to live fully in the present. Its clear-thinking qualities ensure alertness: the ability to concentrate and to be attentive to details You usually possess a good memory, because of your tendency to hang on to everything, but when memory does need a boost of retentive power then this essence also does the job.

Sidetracked.... Helping you to see things objectively, **Bunchberry** essence strengthens the mental faculties, so that you become less distracted by who or what is going on in your environment. It trains you to become less sidetracked by other issues that can waste time and drain your emotional energy.

> *'I am attentive, focused in the present and my thoughts are concentrated'*

Holding on to past hurts

Just as the crab, Cancer's symbol, with its strong claws, clings on tenaciously, so you can find it difficult to let go of your feelings and emotions.

Releasing sadness....

Washing away sad memories and past hurts, the essence of **Sturt Desert Pea** enables you to let go of any old hurts as well as pain which you may have bottled up. Unresolved pain can greatly affect your wellbeing and impact your ability to progress with future plans. This essence resolves these sorrows by safely bringing about the expression and subsequent release of the emotions involved.

Confronting fears....

Putting painful experiences in the past helps you to get on with your life and not miss out on any new opportunities. Confronting your fears when you expect a repeat of past hurts needs the positive and regenerative qualities of **Menzies Banksia** essence. This essence imparts courage, allowing you to move through pain and back into a position of optimism.

Washing away grief....

River Beauty essence has a cleansing quality that washes away the hold of powerful emotional energies. Sadness and grief are replaced with a feeling of vitality and freedom with this essence. It instils awareness that when unpleasant past experiences have been removed, there is rich potential for new experiences and future growth.

Letting go of hurts....

Known as 'The Healer's Healer' (Lila Devi's phrase), **Raspberry** essence is suitable for the Cancerian who is so often the healer and nurturer of others. Being closely involved with others, you can take what they say to you too personally. **Raspberry** increases understanding and wisdom, enhancing your ability to let things go and release past hurts.

> *'I let go of anything that I no longer need as I move ahead unencumbered'*

Nurturing and mothering issues

We all have both a feminine and masculine side to our natures, which ideally needs to be expressed in a balanced fashion. When our feminine side is underactive, it can result in insensitivity and an inability to provide nurture and care for others. When the feminine side to our nature is over-emphasized, it can result in excessive emotionalism, dependence on others and sometimes the tendency to use guilt and manipulation to control people. Cancer is a sign concerned with nurturing, whether of self or others, so this equilibrium is important to maintain.

Maintaining balance....

Goddess Grasstree essence creates a loving wisdom that is understanding and supportive of other people. It develops an attitude that balances your needs with theirs, especially if your tendency is to rely on using emotion to have power over them.

Supplying one's own needs....

It is important for you to feel loved and needed, but some Cancerians can depend on others too much in order to get these needs met. To a certain extent, learning to be your own mother and developing a healthy sense of self nurturing and self-love is a salutary lesson, and helps you rely less on others. *Japanese Magnolia* assists you to become independent and self-nurturing. This essence reduces dependency and increases fulfilment in providing for your own needs and finding inner happiness.

Self-nurturing....

Sea essences are particularly suitable for the watery crab, and **Barnacle** essence lends itself nicely to Cancer types. According to Sabina Pettitt (ENERGY MEDICINE), the keywords for this essence are 'Intuitive, Yielding and Nurturing'. She writes that **Barnacle** types 'will always appear to be seeking nurturing and nourishment from outside themselves'. The nature of the **Barnacle** is to cling tenaciously to the rocks on which it lives, which can be symbolic of the state of dependence. Her affirmation for this essence is 'I embrace the softness within'.

> *'I am comfortable and nurtured by my own self-love and I know that I am able to meet all my own needs'*

Balancing Cancer energy

The Moon is associated with habits as well as feelings and emotions. This means that you can become easily conditioned and fall into patterns and routines, even when these are not in your best interests. Family conditioning can be especially pertinent to you as you are usually very involved at the family level. With your kind and helpful disposition, it is very easy for you to assume the caring role, but in doing so you can sometimes become resentful of, or even exhausted by these demands. You can also become drained by either hanging on to or living in the past. As home-orientated people, Cancerians need to feel safe in their surroundings in order to feel secure, balanced and well in life.

Shifting detrimental conditioning

Cancer's natural instinct to assist means you can overdo the helping and caring of others and end up feeling bitter and hurt when your efforts go unappreciated. One-sided relationships can develop, resulting in your feeling used and taken for granted. Often unable to speak up, feeling that you will be rejected, you hold your feelings in. Your anger and bitterness can then increase, diminishing your sense of wellbeing and your actual physical vitality, and sometimes creating illness.

Feeling un-appreciated....

Helping you to express the truth of your feelings, **Catspaw** essence does not let a situation in which you are unappreciated continue. The effect this essence has is one of changing the energy or shifting the balance in a relationship, so that others involved, knowing how you feel, have the opportunity to respond appropriately. According to their response, you will know where you stand, either experiencing more appreciation from them or, if not, in a position to do something about it.

Feeling over-responsible....

You can often carry the expectation that you should take on more than your fair share of commitments or responsibilities. **Boab** essence is powerful enough to release these unhealthy thought-patterns or detrimental habits. With the assistance of this essence, you are able to make your own decisions without feeling trapped by family precedent and beliefs.

Feeling exploited....

Over-anxious to please, you can be exploited by others, to the extent that you become exhausted and overworked. **Centaury** essence restores individuality, so that you do not neglect yourself or lose your own identity. It enhances willpower so you become less submissive and more your own person.

> *'I release any habits that are not in my best interests'*

Letting the past go and living in the present

The sentimental Cancerian stores both nostalgic and hurtful moments in their memories to be examined or picked over at a later date. This preoccupation with the past is often to your disadvantage; holding on to everything ensures that the past is where you will stay. Any investment required to stay connected to the past takes effort and affects physical vitality, so it is far more desirable to channel your energies into taking advantage of and enjoying the present moment.

Embrace the moment....

Honeysuckle is the essence for those people that hold on to the past, either unable to forget certain events, regretting missed opportunities or believing that life was better 'back then'. Being so stuck in the past leaves you little opportunity for the future, but **Honeysuckle** essence shits the past into its rightful place and encourages you to embrace the present moment.

Change the present....

Judy Griffin (FTH) associates the personality needing to live in the past with uncomfortable circumstances in their present, which they are unwilling to change. She writes, '**Morning Glory** (PF) is the essence that will fire the flame for the future through progressive thoughts, and faith in oneself that change will always allow opportunity for advancement'.

Move on....

Bottlebrush is the essence for all life changes, situations and transitions, as it aids the apprehension or hesitancy experienced during any alteration to your life circumstances. It not only helps you cope more easily with new situations and experiences, it also assists in enabling you to let go of the past and move on.

Focus in the now....

Clearing vagueness and the tendency to escape or withdraw, **Sundew** essence has grounding energies that help you to stay focused in the present—decisive and attentive to detail. It encourages you to earth your ideas, visions and imagination and thus become more inspired to find ways of relating them to the material world.

Home is where the heart is

Security and the establishment of a stable home base are crucial to Cancer's sense of safety and wellbeing. If it is necessary for them to move around for any reason, then Cancer subjects usually have the ability to carry their homes with them, so wherever they are they can immediately create a snug, secure nest.

Home....

Most appropriate for you is the essence of **Hermit Crab**. In view of the name it comes as no surprise that this essence is linked with contentment and peace, feelings very important to most Cancer people. This essence increases ease and satisfaction with yourself and reduces fearful feelings. It helps you to make your home anywhere, and if necessary cope with periods of loneliness.

Creating roots....

If you do find difficulty in adapting to new environments, then *Cow Parsnip* essence imparts a comforting feeling of contentment, enabling you to feel at home in any location. Supporting you during times of transition and when you are unable to settle comfortably in a location, this essence helps to establish a stable, rooted connection wherever you happen to be.

Homesickness....

Dealing with homesickness is a speciality of **Honeysuckle** essence. It heals by dealing with the melancholy and the longing for something that is not available by bringing you into the present moment and regenerating interest in what is available for you as an individual, now.

Hoarding....

Cancerians are typically hoarders and collectors. Their cupboards will probably be packed with food, just in case.... Their homes are likely to be full of possessions with some sort of memory attached to them, memories that make the Cancerian feel protected, safe and comforted. When sadness and pain are attached to these articles it can block the flow of energy and bring stagnation. This in turn affects many aspects of your life, because nothing new is welcomed in. Cancerians make ideal candidates for a Feng Shui 'space clear'. Removing clutter can be a cathartic experience which is rejuvenating and transforming. **Bottlebrush** essence deals with change and will permit Cancer to let go of things that are no longer needed. According to Ian White (ABFH) this essence, taken together with **Sturt Desert Pea**, will help an individual to deal with old hurts associated with certain items.

Releasing....

Begonia essence encourages you to see life without fear or limitation. It helps you to release possessions you no longer need and to embrace new experiences.

> 'I am content with myself and
> I can feel at home anywhere'

Peace of mind

Cancerians can have a tough job attempting to remain untouched by the rigours of life. Easily thrown off-balance coping with life's ups and downs, they can be left drained and lethargic by the events of life.

Coping with disruption....

Narcissus essence has a nurturing energy that helps you more easily digest issues and experiences, bringing about the ability to face challenges without worry or anxiety. This essence works on assimilation both mentally and physically, which helps you to feel safe, centred and grounded in the knowledge that problems and fears can be resolved without upset and disruption to your wellbeing.

Remaining calm throughout disturbances....

Described as 'The Peacemaker' by Lila Devi, the flower essence *Pear* has unshakeable qualities. Regardless of your circumstances, it makes it possible for you to remain composed, steady and centred. Instead of your constantly riding the high seas of choppy emotions, *Pear* can help you feel as if you are gliding across a tranquil lake. Rendering you able to handle disturbances and disruptions in your life, this essence maintains a state of peace and calm for Cancer.

Coping with dramas....

Heart of Peace is a combination of several essences that focus on creating peace and stability. For all worries, traumas and dramas in life, this essence restores balance and proportion, so you are able to perceive life with calm detachment.

Daisy essence provides for the sensitive and vulnerable Cancer, allowing you to feel safe in your own cocoon yet impervious to any confusion, disorder or distractions going on around you. Protective and centering, this essence shields you from overwhelming situations and helps you to stay focused on your purpose. Not only is it strengthening for the oversensitive type, it is for those that are easily influenced to go against their better judgment. Marion Leigh writes that the 'essence of *Daisy* allows us to remain calm and centred amid turbulent surroundings or overwhelming situations, creating a safe space in which to be vulnerable'.

> *'Regardless of what is happening in my life,*
> *I remain composed and unshakeable'*

Relating and communicating

Cancer is usually happiest in a longterm, committed relationship, and probably fits best with a partner who is able to complement their sensitive and sometimes irrational natures with a little objectivity and rationality. Very caring and accommodating of others, Cancer needs to maintain the right balance between caring for him- or herself and not overdoing the care of others. Their extreme protectiveness over loved ones and highly-tuned self-defence system can at times cause some unexpectedly sharp exchanges with others.

Maintaining equilibrium when caring for others

With your tendency to give away too much of yourself to others, it is essential you establish balance in your caring activities.

Wisdom....

Leafless Orchid essence deepens your understanding of exactly what being a carer is. Its supportive energy increases wisdom so you know exactly when to stand back and exactly how much is healthy to give to others. This essence is excellent when you are burnt out, drained or overwhelmed by caring for others.

Boundaries.... Helping to create healthy boundaries between yourself and others, *Pink Yarrow* essence is for the Cancerian who is extremely aware of and vulnerable to other people. It provides objectivity and detachment for those who easily fuse with others and take on their feelings and moods, a habit that can affect them unfavourably. This essence helps you to become more balanced and self-contained, so you create limits that cannot be infiltrated by the inappropriate emotions and the feelings of others.

Revitalizing.... Working on the emotional and mental level, the energy of **Alpine Mint Bush** essence has a renewing quality, revitalizing those people who become worn down by responsibility for others. If you work in any sort of caring position or in the service or welfare of others, this essence is rejuvenating, increasing motivation and enthusiasm in your work.

Objectivity.... **One-Sided Wintergreen** essence deepens your understanding of how your energies affect others. This awareness enables you to give out the type of energy that draws towards you only those who support your highest good. It enables you still to care deeply for others, but only where you are more appreciated and not taken advantage of.

> *'Standing true in all my relationships, I give what I can without jeopardizing my own wellbeing'*

Ditching dependence on others

Cancer's desire to be needed and loved is sometimes so overwhelming that it can smother others. Ultimately this creates imbalance in relationships, as some Cancerians attempt to get their needs met by dependence rather than mutual respect and appreciation.

Neediness.... The wisdom of **Snake Bush** essence supplies inner contentment, where needy feelings are replaced by self-approval and emotional independence. This essence helps you give only when and where appropriate, so that giving is no longer out of balance with receiving and gratitude.

Abandonment.... **Grape** essence focuses on love, healing any neediness or feelings of abandonment in relationships. This essence helps you to feel nurtured and free to love and experience relationships without clingy behaviour, expectations or demands.

Dependence....   For those who find their love is not reciprocated and desperately need love from others to make themselves feel complete, **Mauve Melaleuca** essence encourages an awareness of the love that is within. If you are such a person, then by enhancing inner contentment, satisfaction and self-assurance, this essence helps you to tap into a higher love to be found within yourself, so that you are no longer needy, disappointed or dependent. It helps you to come from a strong base of self-love, where you can see any experience of worldly love as an extra bonus in your life.

Courage....   If you feel frustrated at your dependence on another person but do not have the courage to change this situation, the essence **Red Grevillea** provides the assistance to leave these circumstances. Ian White (ABFE) writes the following about the type of person who can benefit from this essence. 'They are often very sensitive to criticism, which drives them further into themselves. This remedy will help them come out of their shells as it promotes independence and boldness.'

> 'My relationships are free of expectations and
> are based on mutual respect and appreciation'

Lessening overreaction

So responsive to others are you that your sensitivity means you can take what others say to heart. If you take things too personally, you can be crabby; you may react moodily or touchily and withdraw into a hard outer shell as a defence mechanism.

Overreaction....   When your thoughts you are clouded by your feelings, **Raspberry** essence helps transform harmful or negative emotions by instilling wisdom and developing understanding. This essence helps reduce overreaction so that you no longer blame others but take responsibility for your feelings and responses.

Detachment....   **Banana**'s quality of detachment enables you to cope without reacting defensively. Helping you to step back and respond calmly, this essence ensures you do not get caught up in another's feelings or take things personally and so overreact.

Vulnerability.... If you feel vulnerable, tending to withdraw or cut yourself off from others, the essence of **Golden Glory Grevillea** brings a degree of detachment. This essence enables you to enter into interactions and relationships with people possessing the ability to cope with their attitudes or handle difficulties, without feeling exposed or vulnerable.

Overprotec-tiveness.... Your imagination can lead you to be anxious and over-concerned for family and friends. Freeing you up from this worry, **Red Chestnut** essence reduces overprotective and over-caring qualities, ensuring realistic concern and caring for others without going over the top.

'I respond with patience and tact'

Protection from the energies of others

Creating a shield.... You can benefit from **Fringed Violet** essence if you take on the feelings or absorb the energies of others. The qualities of this essence protect you from the potentially negative and draining energies of other people. Helping to keep your life-force intact and balanced, this essence can also be taken after shock, trauma and surgery.

Feeling safe.... **Daisy** essence enables you to maintain sensitivity to others while keeping a calm centre, which cannot be penetrated by the many distractions and demands of other people. The affirmation for this essence is 'I am calm and centred and feel safe in my world' (Marion Leigh).

Inner strength.... The shielding strength of **Hybrid Pink Fairy Cowslip Orchid** essence creates a wellspring of inner strength and resilience. If you feel the feelings of others intensely, this essence acts as a filter so that you become less affected by their emotions and can respond sensitively rather than reacting emotionally.

Defending.... **Guardian,** a combination of several essences, is extremely useful for all sensitive people. This essence protects by surrounding you with a strong energetic boundary that prevents the absorption of unwanted energies. It defends and shelters, so you can feel safe and guarded in your own space.

Stability....

Tomato, a strengthening essence, helps you to remain unaffected by the invasive energies of other people. In addition to providing stability, this essence battles against apprehension and hesitation and instils the courage to tackle fears that have causes both known and unknown.

> *'I am totally protected and remain*
> *unaffected by inharmonious energies'*

Maintaining equality in relationships

Self-esteem can sometimes be an issue for the Cancerian who tries to find respect, love and self-worth by trying to please others.

Feeling oppressed....

Where these sorts of dynamics exist, there is a danger that you can be exploited by others. The essence of **Urchin Dryandra** increases appreciation of yourself and boosts self-respect, thus ensuring that your future relationships are built on healthy foundations.

Feeling disempowered....

The empowering energy of **Monkeyflower** essence moves you into a position of strength, where you are able to create strong boundaries for yourself. Self-assured and full of your own convictions and certainty, you can enter into relationships without inclining to give your power away.

Feeling compromised....

The dignified quality of **Parakeelya** essence encourages self-esteem and assertiveness, thus replacing a thankless 'doormat' consciousness with self-assuredness and awareness of your inner power. Relating can be transformed with this essence, as you find your relationships become more balanced and no longer compromised or unappreciated by others.

> *'My interactions with others are healthy and joyful'*

Resolving possible physical imbalances

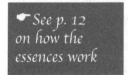
See p. 12
on how the
essences work

Please note that throughout this book suggestions of a medical nature are not in any way claiming that the essences will cure disease, and should not be followed as a substitute to consulting a qualified medical practitioner.

Assimilation and digestion

It is most important for you to keep calm and unruffled, as in doing so your digestive system will operate more easily. *Chamomile* essence and the gem essence *Moonstone* work both on an emotional level (quietening feelings and nerves) and also have a balancing effect on digestive upsets. The smooth, emotionally-calming energy of *Crowea* essence is suitable for all stomach ailments including stomach ulcers. *Paw Paw, Dog Rose* and *Peach-Flowered Tea Tree* essences work on enhancing assimilation of nuitrients and resolving digestive problems.

Essences that benefit sufferers from eating disorders and the emotional dynamics behind them include *Sea Palm* and *Urchin.* The nurturing energy of *Narcissus* is good for the nervous stomach. It addresses worry, fear and anxiety in addition to promoting digestion and aiding with digestive disorders such as excess stomach acid or ulcers.

Sponge is an appropriate essence for Cancer, linking the crab with a fellow sea creature. This essence is good if you are a Cancerian that finds it difficult not to absorb the energies of others—causing you emotional upsets which can affect your stomach.

According to Judy Griffin (THF), *Peppermint* essence aids the individual who is fearful and believing in loss. She goes on to say that when the belief-pattern is one of limitation there is a feeling of lack of control in life. This can result in incomplete digestion of protein. *Peppermint* builds confidence, and its calm energy helps to release blocks in the intestines. She also says that people that need *Moss Rose* essence experience anxiety and a feeling of lack which may result in irregular glucose regulation and poor digestion of starches and fats. See also 'Elimination' in the Scorpio section.

Fluid imbalances

Astrologically, the Moon rules the distribution of body fluids and that has an influence on why some Cancer people are prone to fluid retention or fluid imbalances. The essence *Bachelor's Button* is appropriate for these imbalances and it also aids the Cancer who finds it difficult to release the past. In THE HEALING FLOWERS, Judy Griffin associates fluid excesses with tears. She says that 'releasing the past and the need to hold onto past pleasures and pains will aid the body in correcting fluid imbalances'. She also writes that *Cherokee Rose* essence enhances the balance of the pituitary, pineal, and hypothalamus to regulate menstrual cycles and reduce fluid retention from female complaints'. Fluid retention can also be addressed by *She Oak,* which aids women's hormonal imbalances.

Reproductive matters

Moonstone is the gemstone most often linked with Cancer, so its choice as an essence for this sign is very fitting. Its nurturing, caring energy is balancing emotionally and soothing during the female cycles. The supportive and nurturing energy of *Goddess Grasstree* fosters compassion and balances the feminine aspect in one's psyche. It is suitable for menstrual abnormalities and female hormone imbalances. *Pomegranate* essence is suggested for all female problems in addition to promoting emotional balance and self-nurturing.

5. THE LEO OUTLOOK ON LIFE AND HEALTH

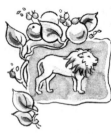

Leo

July 23–August 23

Quality & element:
Fixed Fire

Ruler: the Sun

Opposite sign:
Aquarius

Soul-lesson: Love

CONSTITUTION

THE SUN is Leo's ruling planet, and it is not hard to relate this image to the regal, expansive and radiating energy foremost in the manner of a Leo. Typically, Leos are generous and outgoing, often with gestures that are grand and majestic. Even the more timid Leo is warm and friendly in his or her approach to others. Leos are usually positive, cheerful, and lively and put their hearts into everything they do. Their warmth, kindness, generosity and charming manner makes others feel special. They are happiest and healthiest when they feel needed and others show them affection, appreciation or love.

Implications for health

Leo is associated with the heart and love, and it is often through affairs of the heart that Leos have lessons to learn. Their pride and sense of personal worth can be easily deflated when they experience pain or emotional disappointment; they can take these hurts straight to their hearts. It is important for them to learn discrimination when choosing partners, as at times they do not love wisely, trusting too easily. Often succumbing to flattery, they can be let down by others. It is very important for Leos to feel that they are loved, and when this does not happen it is all too easy for them to carry their emotional hurts and tensions in their back or chest area. It has been suggested in books on metaphysics that becoming isolated from our feelings, feeling unloved, hurt or rejected has a huge part to pay in the occurrence of heart attacks. Louise Hay, in YOU CAN HEAL YOUR LIFE, proposes that those who deny themselves joy and love constrict the heart and make it susceptible to illness.

As this is Leo's area of weakness they need to take care not to 'take things to heart', to cultivate a healthy self-love, to share their love and to accept love from others. If they have suffered rejection in the past, it can deflate their egos and bring a tendency to negativity. If this is the case, it is beneficial that a Leo works consciously not to repress his or her feelings or withhold love and affection from others. In finding an outlet in which to give their attention to others, Leos will find that their own needs are met.

Discomfort manifesting in the back or chest areas is usually a good indicator that they need to proceed more carefully; particularly since, Leo being a fire sign, they can burn themselves out with enthusiasm or overstrain.

HEALING AND SELF-DEVELOPMENT FOR LEOS

The mind

If you are a Leo, you have a strong sense of personal worth. It manifests in a kindly, generous and optimistic nature, and a spirit that positively glows with inner radiance, like a fire that is always burning. You usually have another's best interests and wellbeing at heart, but sometimes you are not always tactful in the way in which you convey this intention! It is in particular the Leo with an overbearing attitude that is not always well-received by others. Believing your beliefs and convictions are best, you can experience upset and hurt when others take your intentions wrongly. Spending some time thinking before you speak, and understanding another's particular orientation to life will help you to understand just how others react, when you tell them (well-meaningly!)

what is best for them! You tend to live more in your heart than in your head, and your main lesson in life is to bring wisdom into your heart, enabling you to encourage and motivate others wisely with love and warmth.

The body

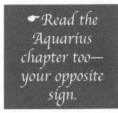
☞ Read the Aquarius chapter too— your opposite sign.

Leo's connection with royalty means that you are not opposed to being treated like a King or Queen yourself. You love the regal treatment, and respond well to the pampering attentions of a health farm or spa. The practice of yoga can develop support and strength in your vulnerable back area.

The theatrical arts are associated with Leo, who has a sense of drama and loves to be the star! The therapeutic use of drama can help you to channel your energies prudently and release your emotions constructively, enabling you to indulge your sense of self-importance and feel that you are getting the attention that you deserve. Leos enjoy having a good time, so your energy is well spent when you are involved in activities involving pleasure, entertainment or sport. What better organizer of such an event is there than a Leo?—someone who will put his or her whole heart into it! When orchestrating and controlling events, you love being in control; you relish having attention and respect from others as this endows you with a sense of grandeur. You are also creative, so it is useful to utilize this talent by applying yourself imaginatively to some project.

The spirit

USING YOUR INNER POWER AND
FINDING YOUR SPIRITUAL MISSION

You possess a huge amount of willpower and persuasive strength, which can be used constructively and positively to assist and encourage others. By directing your confidence and enthusiasm with the noblest of intentions, and not allowing ego or vanity to get in the way, this is where you can manifest your greatest inner power. In pursuit of your

☛ For the
Soul-lessons, see
pp. 13 & 25

soul-lesson of love, your warm Leo personality has much to offer others through support, comfort and inspiration, and by providing them with hope and faith. Leo's soul-lesson includes knowing how to use creatively and direct wisely the power of love (both to others in the broadest sense and personally). Your gift of administration, organization and bringing others together is one area where you can channel your energies purposefully. Often entrusted with responsibility for others, it is helpful to access your inner guidance when deciding what is in another's best interests. As a tower of strength yourself, you are happy for others to lean on you for support, but you must not forget and deny yourself the love and support you yourself need. You will find that helping others will return your own need for recognition and love.

SUGGESTED ESSENCES FOR LEOS

Resolving possible personality imbalances

When we think of the Leo personality, we tend to associate it with the attributes of boldness, courage and confidence. These qualities dispose you well to positions of leadership, where you can manage and direct others. Not all Leos are leaders, but even the more timid Leo likes to be highly thought-of and admired. You feel best and enjoy high spirits when others hold you in high esteem. However, a Leo can become out of step with others if he or she does not possess a healthy sense of inner authority or a balanced ego. Both are necessary qualities in life and essential in providing an individual with a strong foundation.

Enhancing inner authority

The natural Leo disposition is honourable and dignified, but when this manifests negatively then you can become overbearing, arrogant and superior.

LEO (JULY 23–AUGUST 23) · 113

Modesty.... Ian White (ABFH) correlates the essence of **Gymea Lily** with the Sun and the sign of Leo. He says, '**Gymea Lily** can help to transmute into humility the excessive pride and arrogance that can often be found in an out-of-balance Leo'. This essence instils a balanced use of your power and tempers any dominating or controlling behaviour with a more modest approach that involves consideration for others.

Taking the initiative.... **Rose Alba** is an essence of great potency and determination. Strengthening your inner authority, it brings forth a positive expression of personal power. It helps you take the initiative; if leadership potential is innate, that quality is enhanced. This essence addresses not only inappropriate, overbearing expressions of power but also the frustration which can occur if your perceived inadequacies inhibit expression of true personal power.

Respectful.... **Vine** essence stimulates any natural leadership abilities, helping you become wise and understanding leaders. It guides you to respectfully direct and manage what serves the best interests of others. With **Vine** essence, your management skills flourish positively and without arrogance.

Empowering.... **Sunflower** essence addresses authority issues in addition to helping strengthen the link with your higher self, so you are guided to act in accordance with your full potential. It fortifies your sense of being and individuality in the world, and it supports expression of your power and inner identity.

> *'I am humble and modest and treat
> others with the greatest consideration'*

Releasing ego-attachment

Just as the Earth revolves around the Sun, some Leos expect others to revolve around them! Even the less demanding Leo enjoys attention. While a healthy ego-sense is paramount to survival in life, a Leo can become very attached to their own sense of self-importance. Behind an inflated self-importance and superiority, there is often a lack of self-esteem or a fear of rejection. This can manifest unconsciously in demanding behaviour or an insistence to be centre-stage.

Self-validation....

Illawarra Flame Tree essence reduces any need to be in the limelight by increasing your self-validation and self-esteem. It instils a greater sense of self-reliance and increases self-approval, so you are comfortable and confident with youself.

Pride....

Embodying qualities of gentleness alongside strength, the essence *Banana* is known as 'The Humble Servant' (Lila Devi's term). This essence replaces great pride or an over-opinionated manner with quiet calm detachment. It changes self-focus, arrogance, and the need always to be right with qualities of modesty, humility and dignity.

Objectivity....

Woolly Smokebush essence imparts a feeling of self-worth, so that you feel balanced and do not expect that life has to centre on you in order for you to feel good. Providing you with a new perspective, this essence reduces reliance on seeing yourself as the centre of attention. If you have a tendency to exaggerate or create drama in order to draw attention to yourself, this essence reduces this preoccupation and allows you to see yourself with objectivity.

Wisdom....

Encouraging you to leave behind any over-identification with your ego, the essence *Round-Leaved Sundew* assists you, if you are a stubborn Leo, to surrender to a higher aspect of yourself in order to develop and progress. It helps those who resist change because they only identify with one aspect of themselves, and it pacifies those who fear the unknown. 'This essence teaches us how to bring the strength and tenacity of the ego into harmony and balance with the wisdom and guidance of the higher self' (Steve Johnson).

> *'I possess a healthy sense of myself*
> *and I seek no outer validation'*

Balanced power

The typical Leo has a healthy self-belief or assurance. Acting in an overpowering and superior manner can ironically be due to a lack of self-respect. Yet there are other Leos who may feel inadequate and frustrated with their inability to manifest outwardly their sense of self and power.

Confidence....	Creating a mature sense of power, the essence of **Balga Blackboy** replaces frustration and inability to be assertive with a confident manner, devoid of any forcefulness. This essence is also useful in helping you tap into your creative abilities, which are an important outlet in a Leo's life.
Identity....	The empowering essence, **Sunflower**, integrates individuality and identity with your sense of authority. Big, bold and sunny, the physical attributes of this flower share many similarities with the actual characteristics of Leo. The lengthy stem could also be said to be representative of the actual spinal column, which correlates nicely with its ability to provide 'backbone' or moral fibre. Its helpful qualities assist if you are looking for a more balanced expression of your energy and power. Equally it serves those who have a weak sense of their own power and wish to strengthen this attribute. **Sunflower** essence allows you to exude your inner being with radiance.
Graciousness....	Named 'The Confident You' by Lila Devi, **Pineapple** essence infuses an individual with a strong sense of identity and personal power, yet that which is blended with wisdom. The positive outcomes of taking this essence seem to be made just for Leo. A negative Leo expression of pushy, imposing and overbearing behaviour makes way for the dignified and gracious qualities supplied by this essence. Lila Devi goes on to say that the positive expression of this essence is its commanding presence, wonderfully entertaining and bigger than life in manner. Who is this if not Leo? This essence will also suit those who wish to become more assertive.
Good judgment....	A perfect blend of power and gentleness is created with the essence *Sitka Spruce Pollen*. Eliminating power struggles, or the fear of using your power, this essence helps to bring inner authority into full and balanced expression. Empowering you to use your power appropriately with good judgment and wisdom, it also enhances the motivation to act with love and respect for all beings.

> *'I use my power in a dignified and gracious manner'*

A wise Leo embraces new ideas and the opinions of others with openness and acceptance. However this does not come easily to all Leos. In keeping with other fixed signs, you can be quite set and narrow-minded in your thinking, a quality that can alienate you from other people. When your natural pride is out of balance, some Leos can become pompous and intolerant. Considering that Leos are often in positions of leadership, it is important that your compassionate and diplomatic skills come to the fore. Leaders or not, most Leos will want to promote harmonious associations between others.

Compassion....

The flower essence **Slender Rice Flower** enhances understanding and humility in your relationships by promoting flexibility, acceptance and the willingness to listen to others.

Objectivity....

Banana essence encourages the qualities of modesty and objectivity. Rather than leaving you to employ defensive behaviour, it supports detachment, allowing a non-reactive response. It instils tolerance, enabling you to interact peacefully and calmly with others.

Acceptance....

Facilitating an open mind is the flower essence **Date**. An easily-irritated or unaccepting nature gives way to a you that is receptive and welcoming with this essence. Rather than that you view everything from your own perspective, it helps you become accepting and accommodating of others and their opinions.

Humility....

If you are a Leo who takes things personally and then reacts defensively, **Red Quince** essence assists you to embrace the truth of what others say with honour and honesty. Helping you grow from these insights, this essence brings greater self-understanding and increases your self-esteem, so you are able to integrate humility into your relationships with others.

> *'My patience and tolerance enable me*
> *to show great understanding to others'*

Enhancing self-respect

Very sensitive to what others say, another's judgment or criticism is capable of flattening you as a Leo, and you can find it hard to see yourself. You like to be right, and your pride does not make it easy for you to admit defeat or acknowledge that you can be in the wrong. You tend to react defensively to any perceived condemnation or criticism. You can be mortified by the thought of being humiliated.

Self-respect....

If you feel demoralized, then **Goldenrod** essence can increase your inner authority and self-respect. This essence helps you to maintain your dignity if you feel affronted and slighted by others. It encourages you to listen to your own inner wisdom and to assert yourself peacefully.

Self-esteem....

How appropriate it is that **Gold** is often linked with the sign of Leo! As a prestigious and stately metal, it makes a fitting gem essence for such a majestic and proud sign. Not only a great balancer generally, **Gold** essence instils self-esteem, a strong sense of identity, and increases your ability to tap into your creative powers.

Self-doubt....

The essence **Alpine Azalea** is indicated for the tendency to withhold love and compassion from yourself or from others. 'This essence is for those who live in an attitude of conditional self-acceptance. This attitude maintains an imbalance deep within the heart which prevents your vital life-force energies from entering and circulating throughout all parts of the physical body' (Steve Johnson). **Alpine Azalea** helps you accept yourself unconditionally, by clearing self-doubts and boosting self-esteem. This in turn strengthens the flow of life-force energy, bringing the body back into balance.

'I hold my self in esteem and reverence'

Balancing Leo energy

Just as your ruling planet, the Sun, shines continually, radiating life-giving energy throughout the universe, you are usually sunny, bright and energetic. Your fire burns brightly unless over-exertion depletes your energy and dampens your radiant glow. There is a playful spirit and lightness about Leos. You like to have fun and to create on some level, so if these elements of your life are frustrated you can become low in spirits or feel dejected.

Misuse of fiery energy

A Leo can often be identified by copious amounts of enthusiasm, a trait that can be very motivating and energizing for those around you. However, when this manifests as over-enthusiasm, you can be very intense. Some Leos can waste energy by such a constantly zealous and fervent approach either to life or to a certain ideal. This 'over the top' approach can result in exhaustion and burn-out, not to mention boring and tiring those around you!

Restraining.... The essence **Vervain** lessens this overreaction by helping you master self-discipline and restraint. You are then seen by others as high-spirited and pleasantly exuberant, rather than obsessive or fixated.

Re-energizing.... As a fire sign you glow intensely but, prone to excess, you can dwindle away your energy. *Opal* gem essence not only replenishes your creative force and recharges your physical and emotional energy but also encourages balance if your tendency is to fieriness.

Invigorating.... Vital in re-illuminating and re-energizing the worn-out Leo, the essence of *Sycamore* uplifts, restores vitality and re-establishes Leo's light within. If you are depleted and exhausted, this essence invigorates your life-force and provides endurance and the resilience to cope with life's challenges and tests with flexibility and patience.

Restoring.... If your intense driving force pushes you over the top physically, resulting in exhaustion, then *Aloe Vera* essence introduces you to a more balanced output of energy. It draws your attention to consider your emotional and physical needs, together with rejuvenating and restoring your vital life-energy.

Recharging.... If you need more fuel to feed your fire, then **Macrocarpa** essence will provide enduring energy at times of challenging activity or stress. This essence recharges the body when energy is low, in addition to reinforcing your awareness of the need to rest.

> *'My self-discipline enables me to regulate my energies with moderation and restraint'*

Enhancing creativity and self-expression

It is important for Leos to create (and this does not just mean artistically): to leave their stamp or make their mark in some way. A Leo likes to shine. If you are unable to display your talents or demonstrate your abilities to the world, you can feel frustrated and de-energized, which can diminish your inner glow and radiance.

Imagination.... Assisting you in manifesting your creative potential, **Wild Iris** essence boosts your imagination by permitting you to tap into a universal source of inspiration. It teaches you to trust in your own capabilities, so you are motivated to bring forth your potential and let your imagination and creativity flow. It also tackles any blocks or hesitations in sharing your creativity with others.

Belief in ability.... When a lack of belief in your ingenuity obstructs your positive expression, then **Turkey Bush** essence helps renew your confidence and restores enjoyment in your own creativity. This essence helps you to find imaginative and resourceful ways of expressing yourself and helps you feel comfortable and secure in conveying your creativity, however that may be achieved.

New directions.... Finding direction for your creative expression can be assisted by **Orange Honeysuckle** essence. It is useful at such times when you are aggravated, unable to vent your ideas or channel your imaginative energies into creative outlets. It also helps if you feel dissatisfied, needing new directions or openings in which to express your inspired thoughts and energies.

Frustration.... Sabina Pettitt suggests **Hooker's Onion** essence as a catalyst for creative expression. The qualities of this essence underline the theme that 'you are only limited by your thoughts of limitation'. It helps overcome heaviness, inspiring a lighthearted approach, which frees up your creativity.

Sharing with others....

Holy Thorn is the essence to aid expression of your inspired activities on any level. It works by opening the heart, so you can more easily become involved with and share yourself with others. Fear of rejection or repressed feelings give way to nurturing, warmth and true expression of your creativity, with this essence.

> 'My creativity flows effortlessly and
> I express myself with imagination'

Joie-de-Vivre

Essentially fun-loving, Leos have natural spontaneity and sunny, joyful dispositions. Depression of this natural vitality and love of life can sometimes occur, especially if their capacity for enjoyment is denied or their affections frustrated. This can leave Leo feeling gloomy and serious, their energy flattened.

Facing fears....

The essence of **Illyarrie** is made from the Australian shrub *Eucalyptus Erythrocorys,* which has bright yellow flowers with spiky fronds radiating outwards just like the illuminating rays of the Sun itself. No wonder this essence has the ability to regenerate Leos when they are downhearted. It establishes fearless courage, which may have been wiped out by the pain of disagreeable experiences or trauma. If life has cast a shadow over your Leo Sun, the spirit of **Illyarrie** essence helps you to face past fears and take up the task to heal yourself. It encourages your 'Sun' to come out once again and your joyful and exuberant self to resurface.

Inner radiance....

Restoring your inner child, **Lily of the Valley** essence reconnects you with your inner radiance and vitality. Its gentle energy opens the heart to a state of simplicity and innocence, so that you do not look outside of yourself for love or approval. It establishes a position of freedom, where you are encouraged to be yourself without placing any expectations on others.

Hope.... — Another spring flower with the energy to push through the harsh, cold earth to receive the Sun's rays is **Snowdrop** (PAC). The essence embodies the attributes of vivacity and inspires you to have fun. It stimulates enthusiasm and joy, especially where there has been an energy block and you feel that you cannot let go or get moving. It motivates hope, gladness, joy and the liberation of once again getting your head up and warmed by the Sun.

Fun.... — *Little Flannel Flower* is the essence of fun and playfulness, and its ability to establish a carefree mood is useful if you take yourself too seriously. Kicking out over-serious and sombre moods, this essence instils happiness.

> 'I radiate warmth and vitality. My enthusiasm
> and joy support me through all of life's challenges'

Increasing courage

Typically, Leo is courageous, but if you are the more timid lion, you may have insufficient courage to motivate yourself, actualize your purpose or manifest your creative potential. Feeling hampered and blocked, you can then lose your natural spontaneity and enthusiasm for life.

Bravery.... — **Dog Rose** essence creates an awareness of passion and zest for life. This essence implants the bravery necessary to generate all sorts of possibilities in your life, together with encouraging an increased belief in yourself. Confronting fears and addressing shyness or insecurities, it brings you the courage to move ahead with confidence.

Strength.... — The empowering attributes of **Tomato** essence encourages an invincible self-belief. Helping you to feel strong and courageous, this essence enables you to tackle everything with conviction. In addition, it helps stabilize your energy, and centres and focuses you towards success and succeeding.

> 'My Self-belief gives me the courage
> and confidence to tackle anything'

Relating and communicating

People are important to Leos. They treat others well and are always ready to help them. Although their hearts are in the right place, Leos often think they know what is best for others. This presumptuousness means that they can impose their will on others and ignore their opinions. Yet when their own efforts are rejected or they do not feel appreciated, they can be easily hurt and may close themselves off from others. This is hard for Leos, as love is vital for them; without it they are like a flower without the Sun.

Feeling cut-off and unloved

If you are hurt or feeling ignored, you often withdraw to lick your wounds. Feeling rejected and that no-one loves you, you can cut yourself off from others.

Self-approval.... Your strong need to be appreciated and noticed can benefit from the self-confirming attributes of the flower essence **Illawarra Flame Tree**. Instilling a strong sense of self-reliance and confident self-approval, this essence encourages you not to be afraid to reach out to others with warmth. This in turn helps you to feel accepted and acknowledged.

Self-love.... Encouraging compassion and consideration even when you are feeling let down by others, **Pixie Mops** essence helps you face responsibility. Rather than focusing on yourself, what you feel that others owe you and how you should be treated, this essence teaches you to hold yourself in a place of love, which is beyond these feelings. The saying for this essence is 'To rise above the Self' (Barnao). It brings the acknowledgment that others may not always act in the way that you expect but at least you are able to come from a perspective of 'not being or doing as they are doing'.

Tenderness.... Helping to fill up an empty, painful heart, **Pink Cherry** essence provides a knowing sense of unconditional love toward yourself and others. Its loving and tender energy permeates your heart, allowing it to soften and open, so you feel compassion for yourself and others. Clearing harsh and rigid feelings, it resolves fear around loving and being loved and helps you to relate with tenderness and sensitivity. This essence also provides warmth and nourishment for those people who have experienced insufficient mothering.

Keeping the heart open....

Foxglove essence strengthens the heart, helping it to remain open instead of closing down during unpleasant experiences. It expands your perspective, which helps you to meet challenges and to overcome the fear of investing emotionally again in relationships after an unhappy experience. This is how Steve Johnson states Foxglove's message: 'While fear is real, love is bigger'.

> *'I draw upon my own deep well of self-love, which enables me to keep my heart open during difficult times'*

Down with dictatorial and domineering behaviour!

Your enthusiasm to lead or direct others can result in dictatorial, dominating or bossy behaviour. If others find you overbearing, this may jeopardize your relationships with them.

Tact....

The essence of **Willowherb** balances power with will, ensuring you are empowered, but conducting your interactions with others with humility and diplomacy. It balances out any over-attachment you may have to self, in the form of self-important or overbearing behaviour, with self-control, restraint and tact.

Balanced authority....

The essence *Vine* integrates strength and wisdom together with authority, catalyzing a consciousness of wise leadership. This essence helps you to support others and to help them find their way, without using superiority or power to deal with them.

Sensitivity....

Sometimes Leo's eagerness to enthuse others with their ideals can manifest in a domineering manner. If you tend to become a 'know-it-all' and are unable to listen to the thoughts and ideas of others, then this condescending attitude inhibits the formation of harmonious relationships. *Yellow Leschenaultia* essence increases sensitivity and understanding, opening you up to accommodate the opinions of others. It inspires the realization that your insights and knowledge can be increased through listening to others, whomsoever they may be.

Another perspective.... An overly confident Leo can give the assumption that only their ideas or beliefs are best or correct. If this is you, then ***Vervain*** essence gently enables you to permit others their own opinions, without feeling threatened yourself. This essence enables you to see things from a wider perspective, and to be more openminded. It encourages you no longer to try fanatically to impose your strong opinions on others. It accentuates your incredible warmth, enabling you to inspire and give much positive encouragement to others.

Appreciation of others.... Enhancing respect for others and an appreciation of their unique qualities is a quality of ***Yellow Hyacinth*** essence. If you feel that others are not equal to you, this arrogance can arise out of your own lack of self-esteem. ***Yellow Hyacinth*** not only increases recognition of others, it conquers feelings of superiority and increases self-respect.

> *'I keep an open mind at all times and treat others with humility and respect'*

Healing hurts in love

An affectionate Leo, you give your heart and love easily to others, and are happiest when you feel valued, loved and appreciated in return. When this does not happen or when your pride is hurt, you can easily become hurt more deeply within. Susceptible to flattery, Leo can be a poor judge of character, lapping up glorification from others. You relish the adoration. Your own generosity of spirit usually means that you see only the best in others, but in reality though you are sometimes let down and deceived by them. The Leo heart is very vulnerable, and hurt and pain can collect here, impacting your ability not only to give out love but also to receive love.

Self-nurture.... The healing quality of ***Rose Quartz*** essence extends self-nurture and self-love, especially if you have been deprived of love as a child. This gem essence helps replace deep wounds and painful emotional scars with a sense of self-love and inner peace.

Healing....   Another gem essence, **Emerald,** is a heart-cleanser and restorer. Bringing balance to the heart, it works towards healing if unpleasant experiences have led you to block further experiences of love. It quells feelings of fear, especially if you feel cut off from love or from your inner centre.

Abundance....   **Bluebell** (AB) essence also works at the heart level, healing feelings of emptiness and re-establishing trust in others. Its keyword is 'abundance' and it promotes the ability to keep the heart open and to keep giving and sharing with others.

Fear of lack....   The typical Leo would prefer not to be a wallflower, standing in the background and feeling unloved. But if this is the case, the essence **Orange Wallflower** helps to supply individuals with the necessary self-love and self-appreciation for them to bloom radiantly. This essence is required when you feel needy, fearful of love being withheld or when blocking off the flow of giving or receiving love. Instilling a deep inner love that is supportive and reliable, this essence makes you aware that there is an endless source of love within yourself upon which to draw.

> *'I love and nurture myself and I always remain open to the flow of love'*

Approval of and attention to yourself

With a need to shine, Leo wants to be the best—and in so doing to receive validation and recognition from others. The entertainer, the showman and the performer, you sparkle when amusing others and love being the centre of attention, especially when showered with compliments and accolades. If you feel you are not loved or valued by others, your internal spark is dimmed. Learning not to rely on others unduly, and to establish a good sense of self-appreciation and love is essential for a Leo.

Equality....   Rather than craving recognition from others, **Cowslip Orchid** essence permeates your being with a sense of inner contentment, ensuring you do not look for attention from others. This essence instils a quality of self-assurance and self-respect so that you no longer expect or demand interest from them. It encourages you to accept and interact with others in complete fairness, so that you do not feel unequal or ignored.

Expectation.... If you are a dominating Leo, used to being the centre of attention and expecting everyone to do as you wish, then *Gymea Lily* essence can assist. This powerful essence allows you to be your own person, standing strong without expectation of others or expecting to be noticed by them.

Approval.... The Alaskan *Lace Flower* is so small it is often overlooked. Its genus name *Tiarella* translates as 'coronet', and refers to the crown worn by sovereigns (Steve Johnson). An apt essence for the regal Leo, the message of this essence is that 'our true importance is not based on whether we are seen, but on the quality of our expression'. *Lace Flower* essence encourages belief in yourself rather than relying on others for approval.

> *'I appreciate myself and need no other audience'*

Resolving possible physical imbalances

☛ *See p. 12 on how the essences work*

Please note that throughout this book suggestions of a medical nature are not in any way claiming that the essences will cure disease, and should not be followed as a substitute to consulting a qualified medical practitioner.

The spine and the back

Ian White (ABFH) correlates the sign of Leo and spinal imbalances with the *Gymea Lily* essence. He writes how effective this essence is in working with problems in the bones and ligaments and how it is used by a number of osteopaths and chiropractors to align the spine. Other essences that work in this area are *Sea Horse* essence, which energizes the spine, and *Vine* essence, which helps to shift inflexible attitudes that can affect the back physically.

Salmonberry essence embodies the qualities of balance and alignment, not only physically but mentally, emotionally and spiritually. Sabina Pettit writes, 'It is said that every thought we think and every feeling we feel are recorded in the physical. Although the results of this essence are reflected in the physical its effectiveness is due to its ability to erase the originating thought or feeling'. This essence affects the physical body, working on the bones, muscles and fascia and aligning the spine.

The heart

As the heart is Leo's vulnerable area, imbalance can occur here when sadness and hurts arise. The mind recognizes the pain, which can then block the energy paths that connect with the heart, sometimes resulting in conditions such as poor circulation. Essence of **Wild Pansy** restores this connection, so that the energy-flow between the heart and mind is re-established and can circulate freely throughout the body once more.

The qualities of **Rose Quartz** gem essence work at the heart level, healing emotional hurt, and this can have a favourable impact on physical circulation difficulties. The essence *Foxglove* (PF) is indicated when the heart beats out of control or poor circulation is detected. It also helps to attract to ourselves fulfilling personal relationships, and it enhances compassion. Significantly, **Gold** is often linked with Leo, who themselves have hearts of gold, so it comes as no surprise that this precious metal is a heart-healer.

The Australian Bush **Bluebell** essence brings energy to the heart both emotionally and physically, and is said to have an influence on the veins of the body (ABFH). Ian White advises **Waratah** essence for heart imbalances. He writes that this essence is being used in Brazilian hospitals for general heart problems including treating ventricular failure and mitral valve insufficiency.

Stiffness and rigidity

Black Mushroom essence aids the individual who fights change, a resistance that can consequentially manifest in stiffness of the feet, calves, ankles and spine.

Dampiera essence alleviates tight muscles, cramps and spasms, which too can be caused by stiff and rigid thinking. This essence can be used topically and is a constituent of *The Australian Living 'Body Soothe' Cream* (AL), which is invaluable for aches and pains.

Promoting qualities of softness and flexibility, the essence *Dandelion* brings awareness of the mental and emotional issues that can be instrumental in manifesting the creation of muscular tension in the body. It helps to alleviate stress by helping you to understand and confront the emotions that can contribute to this tension.

6. THE VIRGO OUTLOOK ON LIFE AND HEALTH

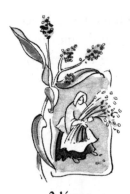

Virgo

August 23–
September 23

Quality: & element
Mutable Earth

Ruler: Mercury

Opposite sign:
Pisces

Soul-lesson: Love

CONSTITUTION

THE SIGN of Virgo is often associated with health and healing, which is not surprising as many doctors, nurses and carers fall under this sign. Others are often drawn to working with their hands in health- and beauty-related fields.

Know for their efficiency, Virgoans are skilled at organization and administration. Their practical natures, together with an instinctive love of hard work, means they know how to get things done. With orderly brains, they can analyze situations in detail and arrive at the most effective and resourceful result. Their eye for detail and desire for perfection means that they are not easily satisfied and can be relied upon to do an excellent job, as they prefer everything to be just right. Virgoans tend to have great kindness, consideration and a natural need to please others.

Implications for health

Virgo's awareness of health and diet can mean that its subjects can be very fussy, with some Virgos adopting fastidious diets or a clinical approach to hygiene. Virgo links with the nervous system, which for them is quite sensitive; their tendency to worry brings nervousness and anxiety. This can be exhausting, not to mention putting pressure on their digestive systems, sometimes causing ulcers, digestive disorders and consequently bowel problems. As Virgo tends to fret when under pressure, they usually prefer working under the direction of a leader rather than taking full responsibility themselves; generally this is more comfortable for them and easier on their nervous systems.

Their discerning natures can make them over-critical, resulting in stress and strain from expecting things to be 'just so'. Quite often hard on themselves, they can lack confidence and fear they are inadequate, which leads them to compensate by trying even harder. Being overly conscientious and seeking perfection in all they do can bring additional worry and tension. Those that stick to strict health regimes can be obsessed with their health, and the destructive Virgo who dissects and self-analyzes compulsively can become a hypochondriac.

Virgo's ruling planet Mercury is associated with the thinking process, inclining these people to approach life primarily from a mental outlook. Their tendency to an over-rational and analytical perspective can mean that they do not always listen, take in or absorb things on an emotional level. This can inhibit the assimilation involved in the digestive process and may result in stomach ailments.

As they are very self-sufficient people, they can at times spend too much time alone, and in their thoughts, which in turn may result in an over-serious or pessimistic stance on life. They can benefit from enjoying the company of positive people to lift their spirits.

HEALING AND SELF-DEVELOPMENT FOR VIRGOANS

The mind

If you are a Virgo, you may be a disorganized or untidy type, although more often than not you prefer to have things neat, and excel at bringing order out of chaos. You are methodical, with a desire for perfection, which are fine qualities to possess, but if your inclination is to be obsessive, they can be detrimental to your wellbeing. Pushing yourself hard and often being critical and demanding, you can all too easily focus on the negative side of yourself or life, rather than the positive. Learning to lighten up a bit and to accept that not all areas of your life have to be perfect all the time can take the pressure off.

Mercury, planet of the mind, can be used to powerful effect if you use affirmations to promote wellbeing, or actually to heal illnesses. Affirmations are positive statements, like those in this book, which when repeated (either out loud or to oneself) can have a potent effective on your thinking, which in turn can influence the physical state of your body.

You are usually found quietly in the background or behind the scenes, serving or supporting others. While this is an admirable asset, your tentative manner often means that by standing at the back you can miss out on life. Participating in some type of personal development or in a course of flower essences may enable you to improve your self-confidence and sense of self-worth. When you are encouraged to move closer to the forefront of things, you can receive the praise you deserve.

The body

You can always find peace by keeping in touch with nature, and walking a dog is an excellent way in which to explore the countryside. You are often the gardener, your practicality enabling you to find enjoyment from growing flowers, vegetables and herbs. Interested in all things natural and unadulterated, you may be guided to choose an organic method for gardening. In your quest for perfection, you usually have the well-manicured garden with the immaculate hedges and borders. It is typical of Virgo to be naturally interested in diet. This can make you a health-fanatic, or at least very selective about what you put into your body. Naturopathy would make an excellent choice for the Virgo seeking help with digestive problems, while herbalism aligns itself nicely with Virgo's thinking.

☞ Read the Pisces chapter too—your opposite sign.

Strongly practical and motivated to work hard, you need outlets that combine these qualities in a pleasant, relaxed manner and enable you to create enjoyable pastimes for yourself, while remaining stress-free. The best choice of hobby or pastime for you is something where your qualities of precision and detail can manifest in a purposeful yet leisurely fashion. You are keen to be doing something useful, and crafts and woodwork enable you to be creative yet productive, and where your application of technical skills and expertise can be utilized. Yoga can provide you with peace, together with the opportunity to position your body with exactness and accuracy, characteristics which appeal to the typical Virgo. Work with your hands such as massage, physiotherapy, beauty treatments and chiropody combines service to others with practicality.

The spirit

USING YOUR INNER POWER AND FINDING YOUR SPIRITUAL MISSION

If you become stressed, hassled, overworked or worn out, you can go off-balance. Born under a mutable sign, you are adaptable, with an alert mind that enables you to understand new concepts easily. It can be easy for you to lose sight of the bigger picture by focusing too much on details, small worries or by becoming obsessed with one aspect of your life. Disconnected from your inner power, you do not operate at your fullest potential. If you are able to take time out to become centred, it allows your strength to recover mentally and physically and for your spirits to be regenerated.

☞ For the Soul-lessons, see pp. 13 & 25

Your soul-lesson is service, yet your overwhelming need to serve in various capacities, together with your tendency to make yourself indispensable, means you can be taken advantage of if you do not use discrimination. Too willing to give to others, you need to learn to give service firstly to yourself. By developing a firm self-image and focusing on your many abilities, you can help yourself not to forget your own mission in life. Learning to ignore your perceived short-comings helps if you can also make others aware of your full potential, your efforts and your contributions also.

SUGGESTED ESSENCES FOR VIRGOANS

Resolving possible personality imbalances

Your natural modesty and unassuming manner means that if you do not blow your own trumpet once in a while you can lose out by being overlooked!

Tackling shyness

Not all Virgos are shy, but your natural timidity and reserve generally mean that you prefer not to be the centre of attention.

Feeling alienated....

Violet essence is useful if shyness impacts your life profoundly and you feel alone and alienated from others. Your tendency to hold back from interacting with people is often because you subconsciously fear you may be taken over or overwhelmed by stronger personalities. **Violet** dissolves this apprehension, allowing you to involve yourself with others, yet still feel protected and strong enough to maintain your uniqueness.

Holding back....

The essence **Five Corners** is for Virgos who holds themselves back, not wishing to be noticed. This essence boosts self-esteem and self-love by releasing a negative self-image and bringing acceptance and appreciation of yourself.

Courage....

Enabling you to express yourself confidently among others is the virtue of **Dog Rose** essence. Feelings of uneasiness subside with this essence, and are replaced with surety and self-conviction. In addition to increasing self-worth, the essence reduces fear and brings courage to go forward in life.

> *'My confidence and courage enable me to achieve whatever I desire'*

Releasing self-doubt

Always trying to live up to the high standards you set for yourself, you are not usually content with yourself or your efforts. Always striving and over-conscientious, you can feel guilty if you are not working or doing something. Lack of confidence in your abilities can push you into working twice as hard as others.

Self-assurance....
Virgos are capable people, but their lack of self-belief means that they do not always think so highly of their own abilities. The influx of confidence delivered with **Larch** essence releases restrictive, self-imposed patterns of self-doubt. By introducing self-assurance, it gives you the opportunity to achieve far more than you realized you could.

Self-respect....
Pine essence instils a healthy acceptance of and respect for your self, in which you see yourself realistically and as fully deserving. With this essence, feelings of inadequacy, guilt and blame give way to self-recognition and pragmatic expectations and goals.

Self-confidence....
According to Steve Johnson, the affirmation for **Tamarack** essence is 'I know who I am and what I can do. I approach life with confidence and self-determination'. This essence helps you become aware of your skills, talents and potential. With increased confidence in yourself and your abilities, this assuring essence will see you through all sorts of situations and new challenges.

Self-esteem....
Snake Vine essence allows you to achieve more than you think you can. Its attributes of positivity and encouragement increase your self-belief and self-appreciation, in addition to renewing optimism and motivation in your purpose. This essence helps you move forward without doubts and without feeling undermined.

> *'I hold myself in high esteem and respect'*

Don't sweat the small stuff

Although good at working with details, you have a desire for perfection, which together with your tendency to focus too intently on the tiny, inconsequential points of life, means that you can waste your energy and become devitalized by minutiae. Swamped by trivia or stuck among the petty, finer points, you can become discouraged and melancholic.

Focusing on the bigger picture....

The expansive energy of **Golden Waitsia** essence encourages you to stand back and see the bigger picture. According to Vasudeva and Kadambii Barnao, the saying for this essence is 'Expanding Horizons'. Giving a spiritual perspective to this essence they go on to say that 'the focus is on the deeper underlying flow of issues not the ever-changing shapes of the waves on the surface'. In other words, it is often more important to have a broader view than to become bogged down with the details.

Expanding your viewpoint....

If your tendency is to dwell on minor problems, the essence **Filaree** can provide an expanded view. It assists you to view daily events and concerns more objectively, which contributes to the effect of reducing tension and anxiety.

Putting things into perspective....

When it is important to focus on the details, yet at the same time still see a situation in its entirety, then **Rabbitbrush** essence can assist. This essence makes it easier to incorporate the minor features into a complete whole, without losing the wider perspective. It promotes a flexible yet concentrated state of mind that encompasses a broader vision, together with the interrelating parts. Patricia Kaminski and Richard Katz write: 'the lesson of the person needing **Rabbitbrush** is to maintain a clear, precise awareness of a range of individual details, while simultaneously extending the field of awareness to include the larger, organizing principles which interrelate the various individual parts'.

> *'I am inspired by detail but never lose sight of the bigger picture'*

Balancing discrimination and sensitivity

As a typical Virgo, you are analytical, which naturally inclines you to scrutinize not only yourself but others, sometimes making you appear quite critical and fault-finding. Some of you are so willing to help others that you can find yourself led into situations that are against your best interests. If this sounds like you, then you are presently learning the wisdom of discernment, and gaining shrewdness in your choice of people and how to determine what is in your best interests. The following essences suit both these situations, bringing about a perfect balance of sensitivity and discrimination.

Objectivity....

Blackberry's positive qualities provide you with an understanding on life that is objective, rather than narrow and picky. It facilitates your having an open, clear mind, so that you can see things as they really are. Replacing any negative or critical thoughts with optimism and the ability to see good in yourself and others, it also encourages you to swap clouded thinking for impartiality and the ability to discriminate fairly.

Discernment....

Snapdragon essence improves your powers of judgment. The advantage of this essence is that it raises one's perception of reality so you become far more discerning, yet in a way that is totally in proportion with reasonable expectations.

Critical attitudes....

According to Ian White (ABFE), those people who need **Yellow Cowslip Orchid** essence 'are focused so much in the intellect that they are often blocked off from many of their feelings. When they are out of balance they have a tendency to be excessively critical and judgmental, as well as aloof, withdrawn and overly cautious about accepting things'. This essence encourages an open mind, accepting of people and ideas, and without the tendency to pass judgment on them unfairly.

> *'I blend discrimination with sensitivity'*

Reducing anxiety and worry

The following essences help release worry and encourage much-needed peace of mind and relaxation.

Calming....

Crowea essence is the perfect choice for the Virgo who has the inclination to worry. Not only does it help to establish a calm centre, it also assists in soothing the stomach. This relaxing essence is ideal when you are feeling stressed, worried or anxious.

A healthy balance....	***Peach-Flowered Tea Tree*** essence removes excessive concern for yourself. If you have become preoccupied with your own health and tend towards hypochondria, then this essence reduces your worrying thoughts and wild imagination. Instilling a more balanced and objective attitude, it also copes with mood swings and inconsistency.
Over-concern....	The expansive qualities of ***Birch*** essence take the Virgo introspective mind away from over-concern, worry and everyday matters. Broadening awareness, this essence helps expand your consciousness so that you are no longer hampered by the inability to see beyond yourself and your concerns. It helps clear any thought-patterns that can hold you back and helps you to understand the inner wisdom of your life and experiences, and so to perceive them in a new light.
Seeing only the good....	Dispelling negativity, ***Wild Violet*** essence releases worry and creates optimism. Named 'The Spirit of Optimism' (Barnao), this essence assists you to approach life without pessimism, apprehension or over-cautiousness. It transforms the unenthusiastic or defeatist attitudes that can cause you to 'miss out' on opportunities or lose chances. ***Wild Violet*** essence helps you to see the best in things and gives you the courage to go into new experiences with brightness, joy and positivity.
Vulnerability....	Over-concern with your health can be tempered with ***Divine Being***, an essence made from *Achillea millefolium* and clear quartz. This strengthening essence encourages you to feel in charge of and able to influence your own health. It creates awareness of those beliefs that can have the power to be reflected physically through illness or disease. 'It reminds us that there is no such thing as "physical" matter. What we think and what we believe is what we create' (Rose Titchiner). This essence transforms thoughts of fear, which can generate vulnerability in the body, with an unshakeable attitude of strength and impenetrability.

> *'I am nurtured, protected and secure in life'*

Balancing Virgoan energy

Often thinking the worst, Virgos can perceive life pessimistically and with disapproval. Worrying too much, together with high standards and expectations, may prompt you to become a compulsive worker. An out-of-balance situation arises when this pattern is to the detriment of everything in your life (especially yourself), and can result in exhaustion or ill-health.

Getting work into perspective

Lack of self-esteem can be a reason why some Virgos feel that they must make up for their imagined inadequacies and flaws by working hard.

Being objective....

When work is motivated by a need to compensate for perceived past failures, **Orchid 'Dancing Lady'** essence helps you to see from a new perspective. This essence enables you to become more content with yourself, as any failures (supposed or apparent) are seen as constructive steps leading to success.

A balanced life....

With a strong work ethic, you often presume that life has to be hard and that in order to achieve anything, it has to come with great effort. The message of **Moschatel** essence is one of celebration and joy in life. Its affirming energy helps you to fulfil your needs by having a balanced life—one that includes fun, enjoyment and self-nurturing.

Reinforcing your own needs....

Willing to help and anxious to please, you can end up doing more than you should, with overwork and often exhaustion as the result. **Centaury** essence increases your individuality and willpower, allowing you to put how much you do for others and give to others in context with your own needs. It reinforces your relationship between willpower and self-determination, so your desire to serve is never to your detriment.

Overdoing it....

Patterns of overdoing and overwork can be addressed by **Vervain** essence. This essence instils self-discipline and restraint, enabling excessive behaviour to be released and a more economical use of your time and energy to be introduced.

Moderation....

Any 'over the top' activity can be aided by **Almond** essence. Known for its attributes of moderation and balanced self-discipline, this essence brings mastery over oneself. Excesses in behaviour or overwork are replaced with restraint, balanced actions and a healthy sense of self-control.

> *'My life is balanced with fun and enjoyment'*

What about me?

It is easy for Virgos to lose sight of their own goals and objectives when they concentrate excessively on attending others' needs or on serving an external ideal or vision.

Your own needs....

Centaury essence instils wisdom, so awareness of your own individuality and convictions is strong. This essence helps you not lose sight of your own mission in life by creating a better balance between others and your own needs.

How much giving...?

If you are a Virgo whose life revolves around catering for or serving the needs of others, then **Leafless Orchid** essence helps you deepen your understanding of exactly what helping and caring for others is about. Its supportive energy enhances your ability to know exactly when to stand back and exactly how much is healthy to give to others. This essence is excellent when you are feeling close to being burnt out, drained or over-whelmed by caring for others.

I am worthy....

Honouring yourself is encouraged by the essence **Cyclamen.** It helps you to see yourself as worthy for attention and consideration. Its caring and nurturing qualities support you by helping you to keep yourself in mind and step away from external demands.

I deserve....

The unassuming Virgo works tirelessly, not usually expecting praise or asking much in reward for their efforts. With your over-emphasis on giving, you can find it difficult to receive compliments when they are due. Helping you to feel good about yourself, **Philotheca** essence encourages you to see yourself as deserving and to accept praise and acknowledgment from others. You deserve it, Virgo!

Don't do it all yourself....

Known for its slowing-down attributes, **Black-Eyed Susan** is the essence for the Virgo who tries to do too much. Helping you to tune into your inner rhythms, it permeates your psyche with calmness and the knowledge that you can achieve, yet in a steady manner. It is also beneficial if you find it difficult to delegate, or are reluctant to entrust others with a task because you feel that you must do everything yourself if you want it completed properly.

> *'I value myself and find it easy to ask for what I need'*

Lightening up and thinking positively

The 'serious thinker' type of Virgo, introspective at times, may benefit from a little lightening up! Your realistic and very practical nature can give you a pessimistic outlook, especially when straining to fulfil obligations, while your strong sense of duty (especially for work) does not always allow for much pleasure, fun, spontaneity or frivolity in your life.

Increasing sense of humour....

Blackberry's uplifting qualities elevate your thoughts and increase your sense of humour. This essence bestows a purity of thought at those times when the Virgo mind might otherwise be closed, judgmental or critical.

Not all perfect....

Your inclination to perfection can mean that you focus too much on your own minor flaws, sometimes to the extent of feeling unclean or impure either in your mind or body. You might feel this even to the extent of disliking yourself or feeling disapproval that you are not living up to some sort of ideal. When this creates an out-of-proportion situation it can add stress to situations and experiences in life, resulting in making you feel infected or contaminated. *Crab Apple* essence addresses this thinking, helping you to keep things in perspective and to realize that you are not always perfect and neither is everything in life. *Crab Apple* can also be a useful essence for Virgo's tendency to absorb negativity; this essence is cleansing and purifying, washing away unenthusiastic or disapproving thoughts. When stuck in details or allowing yourself to be harassed by petty concerns, then it can help you to see things objectively and in context.

Expecting too much....

Virgo's admirable, dedicated and committed manner can often benefit from the lightening up and relaxing energy of *Fig* essence, which releases the unrealistic expectations you may have of yourself. It replaces limiting and critical inclinations with acceptance, so that you feel comfortable and easy about yourself.

Freeing....

The loosening-up qualities of **Rock Water** essence free you from excessive self-discipline, perfectionism or denial of your needs. Encouraging an open mind and a flexible attitude, this essence enables you to enjoy yourself more and take pleasure in life.

> *'My thoughts are radiant, positive and joyful'*

Using your potential and finding a satisfying purpose

You like to be of help and to know that your energy and efforts are employed in some constructive and purposeful endeavour. When you are feeling useful or that you are doing something productive or beneficial, this is wise; otherwise you can feel unfulfilled or frustrated. It is also best that your restless, nervous energy is channelled positively.

I know where I'm going....

If you feel you need to know where you are going, **Wild Oat** essence puts you back in touch with your purpose. It helps you to combine opportunities with your talents and to align them with your true mission in life.

What is my purpose...?

Helping you get in touch with the work you are here to do, **Sapphire** gem essence brings clarity of direction in your life and your destiny. Helping you align your spiritual responsibilities with your actual physical capabilities, its supportive energy raises awareness and commitment to your highest purpose.

What is my path...?

By helping you get in touch with your true self, **Paper Birch** essence increases knowledge of which path is in the best interest of the person you really are. Clearing outdated thoughts and conditioning, its calming influence shifts old beliefs and brings continuity to your actions, so you always act in your highest good.

Letting go of expectations.... Restricted by self-imposed expectations and not wanting to fail, Virgos can be stuck in self-limitation. Going with the flow and trusting there is an inner wisdom in the sequence of your life is assisted by *Hazel* essence. It removes any controlling and limiting thinking, enabling you the freedom to realize your potential and the motivation to fulfil your unique purpose. The affirmation for this essence is 'I travel forward in life with wonder and joy' (Marion Leigh).

> *'I find satisfaction from my accomplishments'*

Relating and communicating

As a quiet, gentle Virgo, you can give the impression that you are self-sufficient and not in need of people, but in most cases this is not true. Your reserved manner can even make you appear standoffish to others, especially as you do not like depending on them and often find it hard to accept praise or favours. You can lose out in relationships by seeking perfection in a partner. Not only can you, if you are the typical Virgo, be conservative with money, you can also be economical with your feelings. Neither are you known for grand gestures—inclining to moderation, you can be often uneasy about voicing your feelings.

Encouraging impartiality

When out of balance, your usual discerning qualities can result in highly judgmental opinions of yourself or of others. Your naturally reserved manner, together with your tendency to criticize, can separate you from people. This may make you appear 'superior', especially as you do not always find it easy to express your emotions. The following essences encourage a balanced approach, enabling you to relate warmly.

Objectivity.... **Yellow Cowslip Orchid** essence reduces your level of criticism and disapproval of others by encouraging you to adopt an objective viewpoint. It supports impartiality, unbiased opinions and increases your ability to give constructive appraisal, which helps you to appreciate and relate fairly to others.

There is no failure....	**Sphagnum Moss** essence helps to impart acceptance, encouraging you to take disappointments in yourself or others as motivation rather than failure. When you feel that you or others are not succeeding, 'never getting it right' or falling short of your high standards, then this essence transforms these feelings. **Sphagnum Moss** helps keep the heart open and promotes positivity in all experiences and situations.
Increasing tolerance....	Intolerant and unaccepting natures can be altered with **Date** essence. Inspiring your qualities of compassion and sensitivity, this essence may change narrow-minded natures. It increases your warmth and sense of receptivity, which encourages others to be naturally drawn towards you.
High expectations....	Those Virgos who tend to seriousness will often see what is wrong in a situation, rather than looking on the bright side or for a positive outcome. This can incline you to perceive life, situations and people rather narrowly. **Beech** essence increases your tolerance for others and raises your awareness, so your expectations of others are realistic and sympathetic. This essence encourages you to become more understanding of the foibles of others, and it imparts openmindedness, so you do not sit in judgment of others who do not come up to your high expectations.
Nurturing others....	You can have high standards for yourself and for others, reacting critically when things go wrong or do not fit with your exacting views. Imbuing qualities of tolerance, the essence **Yellow and Green Kangaroo Paw** enhances your understanding and nurturing attributes, and lessens any sharp appraisal of others. Known as 'The Value of Mistakes' (Barnao), this essence inspires acceptance of mistakes and acknowledgment of their importance as a learning tool.

> *'I reach out to others with warmth and understanding'*

Wounded parties

Willingness to take responsibility can find you taking on more than your fair share of the workload, sometimes to the extent of self-martyrdom. Feeling weighed down and hard done-by at times, you may take on the role of victim or martyr.

Finding support....	Its very name contains the hint that the essence **One-Sided Bottle Brush** may balance your perspective if you are feeling alone, unsupported or overwhelmed by the demands of others. This essence helps you to value the contributions of others, while increasing opportunities for sharing responsibilities.
Equity in relationships....	The essence **Urchin Dryandra**, taken to ensure you are not exploited by others, increases self-appreciation and boosts self-respect. It helps you to move away from any inequality in relationships, especially if you feel inferior, victimized or downtrodden. The dynamics of relating can be changed as you use this essence, encouraging future relationships to be built on healthy foundations.
Personal power....	The essence of **Southern Cross** teaches that we each create our own reality by the way we think and act. Therefore the more optimistic you are, the more you draw positive people and circumstances towards you. The reverse of this thinking is creating a victim-consciousness, in which you continually reaffirm negativity and pessimism and becomes stuck in that mentality and all it attracts. **Southern Cross** essence confirms and implants the message that the universe always gives you exactly what you expect; so if you continually regard life as affirmative, abundant and joyous, then this is the sort of energy that you draw towards yourself. The supporting and encouraging energy of this essence in effect increases your personal power through positive thinking. It pulls you out of victim mentality by instilling the sense of responsibility for your own actions.

> *'My relationships are balanced and I have encouragement and support from others'*

Just say 'No!'

Your accommodating nature can result in your being taken advantage of, so that you end up feeling unacknowledged and used. The following essences help you stand up for yourself.

Being assertive....	The dignified quality of **Parakeelya** essence encourages your perception of self-worth and your assertiveness. It replaces a thankless 'doormat' consciousness with self-assuredness and greater awareness of your inner power. Transforming your way

of relating, it helps you create balanced relationships, where you will no longer find it necessary to bow down to others.

A sense of self....

Lobelia essence works on strengthening your boundaries. If you are easily influenced by others, this essence increases your sense of self and instils determination, so that in decisions you are not swayed away from your judgment.

Your own person....

When your natural ability to serve others becomes unbalanced, you can become easily abused or misused, sometimes to the point of being exploited. **Centaury** essence gives you the power to be your own person and to follow your own inner mission, while still giving service to others in a balanced manner. It encourages your powers of discrimination, allowing you to say 'no' to others when necessary.

Standing up for yourself....

Increasing inner strength is one of the attributes of **Geraldton Wax** essence. It improves self-assurance, so you find that you are able to stand your own guard with this essence. It encourages you not to be so easily influenced or compromised by others. Neither do you bow down or give in, except to what you feel to be right.

> *'Serving others fulfils me, but I never lose my integrity in doing so'*

Increasing personal power in relationships

The modest Virgo who is unassuming and obliging to others does not always express his or her own feelings or individuality in relationships.

Self-conviction....

If you are overly amenable, you can acquiesce too easily to another or give your power away. The empowering essence of **Monkey Flower** permeates your being with a sense of conviction and the courage to express what is in alignment with your highest truth. It enables you to radiate your individual self with boldness and strength.

Commanding respect....

Dill essence can change the power balance in relationships and assist in re-establishing your power if you have given it away to another. It infuses you with an increased sense of personal power that is noticed by others, resulting in a shift in how you are perceived and treated. Rather than being treated as the victim, you are enabled to reclaim your authority and command respect.

Not being taken for granted....

Yellow Cone Flower essence is known as 'The Recognition of Self' (Barnao). If you are feeling undervalued or taken for granted this essence amplifies your sense of self-esteem. The contentment and strong self-assurance it brings makes it unnecessary for you to need recognition from others or to be put in a position where you feel unappreciated.

Not being overlooked....

With a tendency to stand in the background, you may be overlooked, and this can increase your feeling of isolation. *Veronica* essence can change the way that you interact with others, as it helps bring you out of the shadows and increases your receptivity. This essence enables you to express yourself freely without waiting for others to approach you.

> *'I am valued and equal in all my relationships'*

Resolving possible physical imbalances

☞ *See p. 12 on how the essences work*

Please note that throughout this book suggestions of a medical nature are not in any way claiming that the essences will cure disease, and should not be followed as a substitute to consulting a qualified medical practitioner.

Calming the nervous system

You have a sensitive nervous system, often highly strung, inclining you to a level of worry and fret that can adversely affect your nerves and impact your vulnerable digestive area. Equally, when your emotions or experiences are not properly assimilated or adequately processed, this can also result in digestion problems. A nervy Virgo can benefit from the essence *Comfrey* (FES), which assists the nervous system by releasing tension and calming a stressed mind. Addressing nervous complaints, *Aloe Vera* essence is appropriate for someone who is so intently focused on outside achievements that they forget about themselves and become exhausted and burnt-out.

The peace and stability that *Chamomile* essence brings also aids the stomach; it is helpful for those individuals who find that stress and tension create havoc in this area.

Digestive matters

The sign of Virgo is linked with the lower part of the liver, the pancreas, small intestine and the spleen. These organs, involved in the digestive process, are concerned with the functions of a discriminating and assimilating nature, so it is no wonder they can be affected by your attitude to life. An excellent essence that links well with the typical Virgo psyche is *Narcissus*. Helping you to digest experiences and introducing calmness in the stomach, this essence alleviates nervousness, worry, anxiety or obsessive thinking, all of which can produce digestive disorders. On a mental level, the essence *Paw Paw* helps you to make decisions and to digest new information and ideas without becoming over-whelmed. Ian White writes (ABFE): 'Early research has shown that real benefits can be derived from *Paw Paw* essence in situations where quality of food intake is diminished, or where there is illness due to malabsorption of food. It com-bines very well with *Crowea* essence for all digestive or ab-dominal disorders'. In his later book (ABFH), he adds that '*Crowea* essence has a very specific action on the stomach, whereby it regulates the amount of hydrochloric acid being produced'. Raised levels of this acid are a common cause of stomach ulcers, while insufficient levels mean that food is not sufficiently digested and absorbed.

Connecting bowel difficulties with a lack of self-esteem, Dr Christine R Page links diarrhoea with someone who is insecure about their position in society. In this same vein, Judy Griffin (FTH) refers to the person needing *Magnolia* es-sence as lacking self-appreciation and not recognizing their accomplishments. She goes on to say that this type of person is likely to suffer health problems related to poor assimilation of nutrients and proteins. Ian White (ABFH) suggests **Black-Eyed Susan** essence for slowing down. He writes that the people who need this essence may suffer from diarrhoea, as their intestines are in a hurry too.

According to Sabina Pettitt, '**Barnacle** types may be obsessive about sorting things out'. She goes on to say that 'their illness patterns can manifest as an inability to absorb nutrients and bowel dysfunction'. This can be Virgo types, who on the one hand have a skill for bringing order out of chaos, while on the other, imbalances can result in fanaticism and obsession. Relief from digestive problems can also be alleviated by **Moss Rose, Peppermint** and **Bamboo** essences.

7. THE LIBRA OUTLOOK ON LIFE AND HEALTH

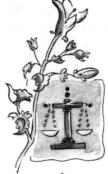

Libra

September 23–
October 24

Quality & element:
Cardinal Air

Ruler: Venus

Opposite sign: Aries

Soul-lesson:
Brotherhood

CONSTITUTION

LIBRA'S sign, the scales, gives an indication that its subjects are learning about the balance they need to maintain in their lives in order to enjoy wellbeing and full contentment. This is not easy for them, because of the tendency of their moods to fluctuate. Charming and amiable personalities, they usually get on well in a social context. As communicators they prefer being with others, rather than by themselves, so spending lots of time unaccompanied or working alone for long periods can affect them adversely. Always concerned with fairness and equality, they make excellent mediators but their idealized view of a perfect relationship or partner is often unobtainable. Tending to opt for peace at any price, they can find it difficult to remain emotionally calm and stable when there is conflict going on around them. Their fine aesthetic judgment and appreciation of good taste means they are often involved in some aspect of beauty or art.

Implications for health

The wellbeing of the kidneys is an important area for Librans to watch. Responding quickly and easily to disharmony, the Libran inclination is to suppress upsetting emotions, yet if they are not careful these can materialize as tension in the kidney area. The tension can be exacerbated when they overstretch themselves, or when they do not face up to any conflict in their lives. If they do become off-balance they can experience headaches, sluggishness, tiredness and discomfort in the kidneys and the lumbar region generally. They can also have problems with their actual physical balance or certain organs or parts of the body that require balance in order to function correctly.

The typical Libran loves to interact with others; rather than being alone, the Libran is happiest with a partner in life with whom to share experiences. Yet it is the area of relationships that concerns them most and which can bring them discomfort if they do not face up to certain realities.

Perhaps Libra's most difficult challenge, the one that brings the most unnecessary stress, is an inclination to indecisiveness. They can easily be influenced by someone one day, only to find their opinions have been changed by someone else the following one. Vacillating between the choices can deplete their energies as well as lose them opportunities. They may also find themselves succumbing to a stronger personality and doing things that perhaps were not in accordance with their own wishes, something which can push them off balance and undermine their wellbeing. Obtaining the correct balance in their relationships and spending time and energy on themselves as opposed to over-concern or over-involvement with others is imperative. It is important that they attend to their own needs and desires, blending a little assertiveness with their great charm in order to actuate what is in their own best interests.

HEALING AND SELF-DEVELOPMENT FOR LIBRANS

The mind

If you are a Libran, you are ruled by Venus, planet of beauty and love. This influence means that you are strongly affected by your surroundings, and appreciative of form, harmony and beauty. Your sense of wellbeing is enhanced by an environment which is aesthetically pleasing; both colour and sound are especially healing to you. However, the whole area of relationships can be fraught with many emotions and fears, which you do not usually find easy to voice. If you are involved in a relationship or recovering from a broken relationship, it is important you learn to release any associated negative emotions, otherwise tensions can accumulate and remain in the kidney area.

Debbie Shapiro writes, 'The kidneys are associated with fear: fear of relationship, fear of expression (especially expressing negativity), and fear of self survival'. It is crucial, therefore, that Librans release their fears and voice their unexpressed emotions.

As a great socializer, you can eliminate stress by balancing your need for relationships with being alone. The more you can take pleasure in your own company, limit your expectations on others and become self-reliant, the healthier both you and your relationships will be. Understanding of others' needs, you must assert your own in order to create a healthy balance in relationships.

The body

It is important you drink lots of fluids to cleanse and flush away any toxins, as this is essential for the smooth workings of the kidneys. Avoidance of a rich diet, instead eating plenty of fruit and raw vegetables, which have high water content, is also beneficial. Just as the kidneys process the waste products that are expelled through the urine, it is equally important that you flush away any negative emotions and habits which can affect the kidney and bladder area if retained. As the whole lumbar region is so key to your wellbeing, you can benefit from massage to this area.

Music can play an important part of your enjoyment and in creating harmony. In this regard, it is interesting that sound vibration is now used successfully in the removal of stones from the kidneys.

As you are so concerned with creating harmonious condi-

☞ Read the
Aries chapter
too—your
opposite sign

tions, it could be of benefit for you to understand and apply the principles of Feng Shui in your home in order to enhance your sense of wellbeing and eliminate any inharmonious energy. Activities that utilize your sense of balance, such as gymnastics, ice-skating, dance (especially ballet), cycling or rollerblading can be therapeutic for you.

The spirit

USING YOUR INNER POWER AND FINDING YOUR SPIRITUAL MISSION

In finding your inner power, you are learning balance and reason. However, many Librans only achieve this state of equilibrium after living through many different extremes, and it is most often through relationships that they learn. Naturally enough, we all choose partners who appear to supply the qualities in ourselves that we feel we lack or we are not comfortable with expressing for ourselves. Especially for you, relationships are a mirror, as you tend to draw towards you those people who can teach you what you need to learn. If you take this to the extreme, though, you may look to others to supply those things that you should supply yourself. You can manifest your inner power when you become your own best authority and when you are in command and in control of your best interests.

Working primarily on a mental level, you are mainly concerned with communications on a one-to-one level. Yet it is in the arena of relationships that your need for harmony is often tested, as you can have much to learn from those whose outlook is in complete contrast to your own. Relationships are also a place where you can explore your soul-lesson of brotherhood. Here you can use your natural negotiating skills, tact and diplomacy to bring unity and agreement between others. Suited to the role of the peacemaker, you make an excellent counsellor; skilled at arbitration, you can bring balance and harmony between opposing factions.

☞ For the
Soul-lessons, see
pp. 13 & 25

SUGGESTED ESSENCES FOR LIBRA

Resolving possible personality imbalances

If your need for other people causes you to depend too much on them, then you must take care to maintain your own identity, be true to yourself and develop your own resources to cope alone when necessary. Make sure that you pay attention to your own individual needs, and then you will be less likely to look to others for approval or acceptance. As a Libran, you can be a mixture of contrasting traits. Not wanting to hurt others, you generally refrain from arguments, but you do enjoy a good debate, the objective of which is usually to reach an impartial decision. Inevitably at one time or another the scales tip to one extreme, and then as you seek to redress the balance you can become involved in quarrels and arguments.

Attention to one's own needs

Typical Librans prefer to spend their lives with a partner rather than alone, but when this is taken to extremes it can result in too much dependence on others.

Independence....

Happy Wanderer essence instils in you self-assurance and independence, giving you the confidence to do things alone and supporting you to stand on your own two feet. Encouraging you to achieve in your own right, this essence brings confidence and belief in yourself.

Courage....

The essence of **Dog Rose** brings the courage to stand up for yourself. It also deals with fear on any level. Particularly, for Libra, this can be fear of being in a relationship or fear of not being in one.

Liberation....

The Libran's nature is essentially concerned with unity and with the maintaining of relationships, so understandably you can find it difficult to extricate yourself from an unhappy relationship. The energy of **Red Grevillea** essence gives you the strength to move from any stuck position. This essence is also liberating if you become too reliant on others or dependent on their opinions and advice.

Conviction....	Self-assurance and assertiveness are the qualities of **Monkey Flower** essence. It helps empower you in order that you manifest your inner convictions. Replacing apprehension or hesitancy with purpose and surety, this essence helps you to express yourself and to act in accordance with whom you truly are.

> *'I rely on myself and achieve in my own right'*

Coping alone

Sharing is far more important to you than going it alone and you are happiest when you have companionship, love and attention from others. Inevitably the ups and downs of relationships mean that it is in your best interests to know how to sustain yourself emotionally in order to cope with being alone when necessary.

Inner strength....	For those times when you do not have the support and assistance of a partner, **Wild Cyclamen** essence provides nurturing and support. Encouraging inner strength and self-sufficiency, it enables you to seek your own counsel and to have the confidence to make your own decisions.
Inner support....	The affirmation that Marion Leigh has written for **Lime** essence resonates with the Libran psyche. 'I open my heart to create harmonious relationships in life. I am one with all other beings'. The supporting energy of **Lime** infuses you with love and lightness, which releases any loneliness and overcomes the fear of separation from others. Instead of feeling cut off or powerless, this essence encourages a 'collective consciousness', which helps you to focus on creating harmony and peace with others, whatever their circumstances.
Inner contentment....	In addition to increasing feelings of ease and personal satisfaction, the essence of **Hermit Crab** instils feelings of peace and contentment with your own company. It eases 'alone-ness' and helps you to cope with any periods of loneliness.
Inner reliance....	The self-reliance essence, **Illawarra Flame Tree,** helps if you feel you need to have other people around you, or if you feel rejected because you don't. Releasing you from the need to

seek approval from others, this essence provides strength and confidence, together with the commitment and responsibility to develop your own potential.

> *'I am content with myself and I appreciate my own company'*

Being true to yourself

Clearing away any inconsistencies and encouraging you to uphold high personal honour, the following suggested essences help you to maintain strong personal integrity, inner strength and resolve.

Self-worth.... The centering and decisive qualities of **Strawberry** essence link well with the Libran attributes. Lila Devi sees the individual benefiting from this essence as a connoisseur of beauty, with the ability to see beauty everywhere, in everything and everyone including themselves. This essence boosts your sense of self-worth, so that you do not have to look to others for approval. It enhances the ability to handle all relationship difficulties, and is helpful in transitions, such as when you are dealing with relationship break-ups. She writes that the dominant qualities in **Strawberry** type people are courtesy, elegance, naturally refined tastes and gracefulness. This relates nicely with the typical Libran attributes.

Being oneself.... Librans can sometimes project a face that is not necessarily true of themselves. Adapting to whatever others expect them to be, or to suit some circumstance that will ensure their advancement or acceptance, they can put on a facade. If this is you, then **Rabbit Orchid** essence releases the masks and allows you to be your true self. Removing the fear of just being yourself, this essence fosters qualities of openness, honesty and truth, which has the effect of drawing toward you relationships where you are loved for just being you.

Standing strong.... The strength of **Cattail Pollen** essence supports you in projecting a strong sense of yourself out into the world, especially when difficulties and barriers impede your progress. It enables you to remain resolute and to stand strong for what is in your highest good. You will also find the energy of **Cattail Pollen** helps you attract the harmony and support of others that resonate at this same level.

Self-trust....

The gem essence **Pyrite** helps Librans to be true to themselves, especially when they need extra strength to maintain their position. This essence not only hardens your resolve, it also promotes trust in yourself and the ability to stick to your decisions and stand up for yourself. When you are no longer influenced or persuaded against your values, it helps you to create only relationships that are in line with your true self.

> 'My truths are honesty and fairness and I always attract these qualities in others'

Calming argumentative natures and overreactions

When one side of the scale dominates in debate, the normally charming, peaceful and fair-minded Libran can show a confrontational and argumentative side to the personality.

Perspective....

Instilling objectivity and a sense of perspective, **Banana** essence helps you to step back and observe a situation before becoming emotionally involved. Coping with quarrelsome moods, this essence introduces clarity, so that reactive dispositions submit to clear thinking, good listening and consideration for others.

Understanding....

If you become clouded by emotion, then **Raspberry** essence helps transform harmful or negative emotions by infusing wisdom and increased understanding. This essence reduces overreaction. You become inclined not to blame others but to take responsibility for your own feelings and responses.

Observation....

Helping you detach, pause and observe before reacting, the essence **Physostegia** encourages you to respond appropriately and peacefully when agitated or perturbed by what is going on around you. It helps you keep calm, centred and unaffected by interactions with others or situations that would normally have distracted or disturbed you. It helps you stand tall and stay centred, especially when overwhelmed by forceful personalities.

Wholeness.... **Macrozamia** is a 'harmonizer', bringing wholeness and unifying the appropriate balance of male/female energy within everyone. It addresses a confrontational attitude, one that is quick to retort in an aggressive manner to a perceived threat.

> *'I respond calmly, appropriately and peacefully'*

Balancing Libran energy

As your symbol, the scales, depicts, much of your life can be spent swinging back and forth between extremes. As they learn about balance, the behaviour of some Librans can be erratic and unconcentrated. The scales dip from side to side until the person learns to maintain a poised central position. Being very objective in your reasoning and always appreciating another's viewpoint means that you do not find it easy to commit yourself in decisions. Not wanting to upset anyone, you can have problems aligning yourself with any one side in an argument. You can change your mind according to how the argument goes, which can be taxing and draining for all.

Holding the balance

Inner poise.... If you are prone to inconsistent moods, ones that constantly swing back and forth, the essence of **Scleranthus** can restore equilibrium and help you find your true inner rhythm. With this essence fluctuating moods, as well as vacillating and wavering thoughts, give way to balance and inner poise.

Standing firm.... **Bell Heather** essence not only restores purpose and direction if you are undecided and lacking conviction, but it also settles moods that swing and natures that are easily swayed. It embodies the qualities of faith and trust, and inspires self-confidence and inner knowing—so you are reminded to stand firm and stable, unaffected by circumstances, trauma, stress or conflict.

Stability.... Capable of handling Libra's up-and-down moods, **Chamomile** essence generates stability. It increases emotional objectivity, so your emotions do not sway from one extreme to another, and it decreases moodiness, thus creating a sense of peace.

Centred....

The key words for **Ox-Eye Daisy** essence are 'Total perspective; for being centred' (Sabina Pettitt). This essence moves you into a still, safe, peaceful centre where you are able to get a greater perspective on things. Helpful for those who can become overly mental in their attunement and spend too much time weighing up the pros and cons, this essence enables you to see the bigger picture and obtain a balanced understanding.

> 'My whole being is centred, balanced
> and in perfect harmony'

Maintaining peace

Obtaining peace in the outside world is not always an easy option for anyone, yet alone peace-loving Libra. The following essences help you to achieve this.

Calm....

If you find it difficult to be emotionally stable when surrounded by discord, the essence of **Rose Cone Flower** provides a safe inner space, where disturbed and edgy feelings give way to ease and calm. This essence enables you to find a peaceful place within, without having to have your external surroundings and circumstances just right.

Harmony....

Scottish Primrose essence restores stillness when your peace is threatened in some way or if there is conflict in your relationships. It returns you to a place of equilibrium and inner harmony, replacing anxiety, shock, fear, discouragement and quarrelsome states with steady, centred energy and peace of mind.

Tranquillity....

Replacing inner turmoil with tranquil feelings, the essence of **Verbena** creates a sense of inner peace. Its meditative qualities restrain impetuosity and rash behaviour, encouraging your body to be relaxed and your mind to be kept calmly in the present.

Relax....

Regardless of what is happening around you, the sea essence **Sponge** enables you to relax and maintain your peace. Sabina Pettitt's affirmation for this essence is 'everything is unfolding in perfection; nothing happens to me without my consent'. Helping to release any impurities from the mind, it also transmutes negative energies absorbed from others.

> 'My environment is always peaceful and serene'

Enhancing decision-making

There is nothing like indecision and procrastination to bring frustration and drain your life-force. Continual swings back and forth can unbalance your fine qualities of impartiality and objectivity, resulting in confusion and delaying decisions and tasks.

Decisiveness....

Scleranthus essence encourages a state of calmness and certainty. It enables you to concentrate your energies, yet at the same time remain flexible and adaptable. It can empower you to consider all possibilities yet make decisions wisely. Restoring a sense of inner balance, *Scleranthus* essence not only helps you to act decisively, it also calms changeable, restless and unfocused energy.

Patience....

When decisions need making, the essence of **Hairy Yellow Pea** provides the necessary patience to cope with these times, without feeling pressured. This essence supports a holding pattern, enabling you to step back from anxiety and worry and to wait until all the relevant pieces are complete in the jigsaw before making a decision. This is very important for Librans who, not wishing to upset anyone, need to raise their minds above everyday concerns in order to reach a point of balance in their thinking. When understanding and deeper assessment of a situation is complete, then you may have the wisdom to act in full knowledge of the choices.

Certainty....

Lila Devi writes about the positive outcome of taking **Lettuce** essence, that it 'also offers the antidote to an indecisive mind: inner certainty. Remove the anxiety, fear and attachment to the outcome of a decision, and you have an individual with all the knowledge—or the ability to gather it—needed to resolve most any problem'. In addition to bringing decisiveness, it instils patience, concentration and enhances your communication abilities by ensuring you speak up for yourself and express yourself in a clear, sure manner.

Empower-ment....

The decisive energy of **Pipsissewa** essence dissolves the anxiety around decision-making so that you are empowered to make the right choices. Sometimes in making a decision you are unable to see the bigger picture and things do not always turn out as you think. In these circumstances, the wisdom of **Pipsissewa** helps you move from a dissatisfied and confused state to one of knowing which moves to make next.

> *'My thinking is clear and my actions*
> *are certain and decisive'*

Just keep going

Usually you are directional and action-orientated, but this can alternate with periods of lethargy and uncertainty. The laid-back Libran is sometimes referred to as lazy, but people can take as laziness your tendency to delay getting on with something until you have reached a decision. At times when indecision overwhelms you or confusion prevails, you can become aimless and apathetic, not to mention depleted in energy.

Motivation.... Perseverance and commitment to keep going is enhanced with the essence **Kapok Bush**. This essence brings persistence when your energy takes a dip, or you become halfhearted and apathetic. If exhaustion is prompted by a discouraged and resigned attitude, then **Kapok Bush** essence restores vitality and motivation when your incentive and enthusiasm are lacking.

Completing.... Wavering and hesitating behaviour is addressed with *Jacaranda* essence. The decisive, clear-minded qualities of this essence replace any dithering, which is so draining. This essence is also for distracted individuals who scatter their energies and do not complete projects.

Resolving.... Marion Leigh's affirmation for **Sea Pink** essence is 'I unite all energies within my being and welcome the balance and harmony'. This essence pulls all aspects of your being into a functioning whole. Resolving splits and balancing conflicting characteristics, it stabilizes the energy-flow in your body.

Stabilizing.... Providing emotional balance and vitality, the essence of **Peach-Flowered Tea Tree** brings stability to mood swings. This essence helps to stabilize blood-sugar levels, which thus provide consistent, stable energy. Its persevering energy helps when lack of commitment hinders completion of tasks.

> *'I am stable and united on all levels'*

Relating and communicating

Venus, planet of love and relationship, rules both Taurus and Libra. Both signs are concerned with the arts, beauty, and harmony. In airy Libra, sensual Venus expresses herself more mentally than in earthy Taurus. This means that the Libran temptation can be to live in an idealized world of thought and back off from powerful feelings and passionate emotions.

Libra is strongly motivated by justice and harmony, but when these qualities are unbalanced its subjects can be misled into using others to benefit themselves. Librans naturally gravitate towards others, and it is in relationships and interactions with others that they will meet most of their challenges, and where they will be working on their soul-lesson of brotherhood.

Communicating with justice and sincerity

Librans' charming and agreeable manner makes it very easy for them to talk anyone into anything! When these attributes are taken to the extreme, the delightful yet persuasive Libran can sometimes resort to subtle manipulative techniques, seeking relationships for personal gain, in order to take advantage of others or to look after their own interests.

Sincerity....
Pale Sundew essence purifies the heart, awakening your consciousness to any controlling and manipulative behaviour you may have embarked upon. It awakens those parts of your psyche that need light and reveal to you your motives, so that deceptive tactics, shallow feelings or insincere deeds are exposed, transformed and replaced with sincerity and genuineness.

Fairness....
Known as 'The Spirit of Fairness', **Swan River Myrtle** essence instils positivity and fairness. This essence is for either the victim or perpetrator of injustice—for a person suffering injustice but equally for a person who lacks the quality of fairness in their dealings with others. Vasudeva and Kadambii Barnao say that it is 'the essence to manifest a non-compromising attitude towards fairness both within ourselves and from others'.

Truth....

The key words for **Easter Lily** essence, according to Sabina Pettitt, are truth, purity, integrity and honesty. This essence is about expressing your true being without having to play a role, put on a mask or use duplicity in your words. If you are the type of Libran who can sometimes be flippant or superficial, this essence inspires your respect for others.

Integrity....

Unifying thoughts, words and deeds, the essence **Fuchsia Grevillea** encourages you to communicate with integrity, prompting you to swap artificial, dishonest or hypocritical traits for truthfulness and openness. Instilling a sense of honesty, it ensures that interactions with others are straightforward and truthful.

> 'My interactions with others are sincere and fair'

Coping with conflict

With their maxim 'Peace at any Price', some Librans can find it difficult to express what is important to them. Preferring to keep quiet rather than upset the status quo, they often accept this deal as an inevitable part of maintaining their much-needed peace. Easily battered by conflicts, most Librans would rather not argue with anyone.

Firmness....

Helping to bring forth a balanced, assertive manner, the essence of **Balga Blackboy** promotes self-assurance. It brings forth firmness in your interactions with others, yet a firmness that is totally in keeping with your naturally tactful manner. This essence also promotes your awareness and consideration of the needs of others, while at the same time breeding assertiveness in your achievement of goals.

Directness....

Vasudeva and Kadambii Barnao write that those likely to benefit from **Start's Spider Orchid** essence are 'those wanting peace and therefore not dealing with difficult issues in a straightforward manner'. This can be typical Libra. Rather than confronting upsetting issues or situations, you tend to compromise or avoid them, which often leads to frustration and upset. This essence can assist Librans in all their dealings with others, providing them with the directness and courage to act decisively and wisely.

**Deter-
mination....**

With your intense dislike of conflict, you find it hard to remain emotionally stable when surrounded by discord. You can often give way to, or adapt to, stronger characters; you may sway to their opinions. The supporting essence of *Pink Impatiens* encourages you to have the courage to stand by your own beliefs and the determination to do whatever you feel is right. It brings great strength in the face of feeling overwhelmed, unsupported or dealing with great challenges.

> *'I cope with conflict with courage and diplomacy'*

Increasing objectivity and clarity

Good in situations requiring tact, Librans make wonderful diplomats and negotiators. Yet when your natural tactful qualities are out of balance you can lose the middle ground. If relationship issues overwhelm you, it becomes confusing and difficult for you to see things in perspective.

Clarity....

Purple Eremophila essence brings clarity of mind, enabling you to separate emotions from the issues at hand. The calm, objective qualities that this essence instils help you not become too emotionally involved. Enhancing your diplomatic skills, it enables you to handle concerns with natural tact and discretion.

Detachment....

Improving your ability to mediate and settle disputes, *Yellow Cowslip Orchid* essence increases your ability to grasp the facts of a situation quickly and help you consider all information compassionately. It enables you to be detached from issues, allowing objective, fair appraisal, and evaluation with unbiased judgment.

**A fresh
viewpoint....**

The essence *Purple and Red Kangaroo Paw* amplifies your understanding of others and inspires you to act with sensitivity and openness in all your interactions. This essence diffuses deadlock situations where each person needs to win an argument or when one of them places all the blame onto another. It encourages understanding from a greater level than the personality and prompts you to embrace a situation from a far more open and unselfish perspective. This in turn gives rise to different perspectives and fresh viewpoints.

Unifying....

The essence of **Harvest Lily** supports the ability to see and appreciate another's point of view. The unifying energy of this essence stimulates the harmonious qualities you have in negotiating and resolving tensions and uniting opposing groups.

> 'I handle all issues with clarity and objectivity'

Resilience in your interactions with others

Inevitably the relationship arena can bring conflicts and disputes, so Librans needs to keep their own space and be strong in their interactions with others.

Enhancing social skills....

Ideal for Libra, the essence of **Queensland Bottlebrush** is known as 'The Sociable Spirit' (Barnao). Strengthening your social skills, this essence enables you to interact with ease, without being drained by the energies of others. It also readdresses the balance when you use relationships for your own benefit rather than for the enjoyment of interaction.

Independence....

Hematite essence provides emotional protection by reinforcing your energetic boundary, which is very necessary if you are the Libran who can consider the other person too much. This essence strengthens, so you do not easily get drawn into others' issues, and through it you are better able to maintain your own individuality and independence within a relationship.

Composure....

As a sociable 'people-person', you may find that your life centres around others. Helping you keep composed and calm in all interactions with others, the essence of **Pink Fairy Orchid** essence instils resilience and enables you to be unaffected by what is going on externally. It generates anew that quiet inner space where you need not react to disharmony or disagreeable conditions.

Protection....

In addition to creating a strong sense of the self, the balancing essence of **Yellow Pond Lily** helps you to feel centred despite emotional issues and attachments that can weigh you down. Liberating you from relationship matters and emotional dramas, you feel protected and strengthened with this essence.

Restoring.... A unique characteristic of the Alaskan *Sweetgale* shrub is its ability to produce, on the same shrub, male flowers one year and female flowers the next. The symbolism of this male/female relationship links nicely with the attributes of cooperative Libra. In regard to the essence's ability to improve the quality of emotional interactions in male/female relationships, Steve Johnson has this to say: '*Sweetgale* helps us reclaim our emotional space after an argument or upset, and restores calm and strength to our emotional centres. From this point of balance we are able to respond more directly and appropriately to each other, regardless of the situation'.

> *'I keep my inner space and I am unaffected by others'*

Being comfortable with feelings and emotions

With a tendency to live more in the intellect rather than the senses, the airy Libran can sometimes find it hard to relate closely. Generally you are happiest with a partner with whom you can communicate on a mental level, one who does not put excessive demands on you emotionally.

Emotional closeness.... If you find yourself going from one relationship to another, or find it difficult to dedicate yourself to a relationship, the essence of **Wedding Bush** promotes commitment. Helpful for bonding in partnerships, this essence helps you to be devoted, particularly if you often run away from emotional closeness. It also helps in achieving your goals.

Commitment.... **Archduke Charles** essence enhances intimacy, allowing you to feel safe when touched. This essence is also for those individuals who put up barriers to closeness or avoid total commitment.

Sharing feelings.... An essence that encourages expression and sharing of your feelings, and comfort around physical closeness, is **Flannel Flower.** Ian White (ABFE) writes, 'it helps people express their feelings verbally and develop sensitivity and gentleness in touching, whether in a sexual or sensual way'. It is also helpful in establishing healthy boundaries for those people who are too amenable with others and have difficulty in saying 'No'. An essence combination that stimulates the qualities vital in all

Expressing emotions....

aspects of relationships is the **Australian Bush Relationship Essence**. This combination helps to improve communications by releasing blocked emotions, and clearing pain and resentments.

Enhancing your capacity for intimacy, the essence **Balsam** increases warmth and sensitivity. Not only instilling love and nurturing of yourself, this essence boosts your feelings, sensuality and warmth towards others, something which naturally promotes bonding and harmony in relationships,

Increasing warmth....

> *'I express myself easily with warmth and feeling'*

Resolving possible physical imbalances

☛ *See p. 12 on how the essences work*

Please note that throughout this book suggestions of a medical nature are not in any way claiming that the essences will cure disease, and should not be followed as a substitute to consulting a qualified medical practitioner.

Maintaining fluid balance in the body

The positive keywords for **Macrozamia** essence are 'balance and equilibrium' (Barnao). Helping to restore physical balance to the water element in the body, this essence also balances and harmonizes the masculine and feminine forces within yourself. The Australian Bush essence **She Oak** has a hydrating effect on the body in addition to treating hormonal imbalances. The sea essence **Brown Kelp** is also helpful in controlling the storage of water and maintaining adequate reservoirs of bodily fluids.

The kidneys

It is important for Librans to keep their bodies hydrated, as kidney stones can develop through dehydration. Debbie Shapiro writes that stones 'can occur when we are holding on to old thoughts or attitudes that should have been released, or past sadness (tears) now taking form'.

Sabina Pettitt has several sea essences among her 'Pacific Essences' that work on the kidneys, the adrenals and the fluid balance in the body. She recommends the sea essence *Surfgrass* for kidney stones and inflammatory conditions. Linking with Libra's essential qualities of balance and harmony, this essence affects homeostasis within the body, mind, spirit and emotions. It stabilizes the adrenal glands and creates a more balanced output of the adrenaline released during stressful and fearful times. Sabina Pettitt also recommends the sea essence *Coral* 'to support the role of the kidneys to cleanse the blood and detoxify the system' and *Sponge* essence to help 'filter impurities from our minds and help to maintain our own energy reserves and fluid balance'. The Australian Bush Flower essence *Dog Rose* is beneficial for all fears and it has a draining and stimulating effect on the kidneys.

Maintaining equilibrium

Intimately connected to your wellbeing, balance is crucial for you to maintain. Problems with equilibrium can manifest as travel sickness or difficulties with actual physical balance. The balancing qualities of *Scleranthus* essence treats travel sickness and *Brown Kelp* essence resolves fluid imbalances in the ears, which can affect one's balance.

Jacaranda essence possesses centering qualities for the personality that either rushes around excessively or dithers and scatters energy. It restores focus, clear-headedness and balance. *Bush Fucshia* essence helps one to become in tune with the rhythms of the earth, and according to Ian White (ABFH) this essence 'is used to successfully treat the following conditions: tinnitus; vertigo; travel sickness; and sense of balance'.

The planet Venus rules the venal portion of the circulatory system and suggestions for essences that benefit this system can be found under the sign Aquarius, which rules the circulation in general.

8. THE SCORPIO OUTLOOK ON LIFE AND HEALTH

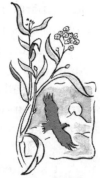

Scorpio

October 24–
November 22

Quality & element:
Fixed Water

Rulers:
Mars & Pluto

Opposite sign:
Taurus

Soul-lesson: Peace

CONSTITUTION

PROBABLY the most intense sign of the zodiac, Scorpio has huge determination and great willpower. A Scorpio is a good person to have on your side! They possess great loyalty and a powerful energy that can move mountains if necessary. Despite having very deep feelings, Scorpio subjects are good at keeping their strong and passionate emotions well-hidden. Beneath their façade they can be hiding some fierce and turbulent feelings. Extremely shrewd, their sharp minds are capable of penetrating to the core of any situation or problem. Scorpio people are very receptive to the energies of other people and their keen insight enables them easily to perceive and understand another's nature, feelings, needs and motivations. This awareness of energy on a subtle level means that they can be adept at using the emotional energies of others. This can range from the self-seeking Scorpio who will use the resources of others to meet his or her own ends to the higher 'Eagle' manifestation of Scorpio, a person who can regenerate negativity and illness in another through his or her own healing strength.

Implications for health

Subjects of all the water signs can hang on to emotions, feelings or situations. Scorpios do this not only because of their dislike and resistance to change but because most of them

like to be in control of a situation. Their inability to release feelings and thoughts can inhibit the natural process of
elimination in the body. This is a crucial factor in maintaining good health, particularly as Scorpio rules the areas of
the body concerned with elimination, such as the bladder,
urethra, colon and rectum. In addition, Scorpio rules the
parts of the body concerned with sexuality and reproduc-
tion. It is important that Scorpios are aware of these vulnerable areas in themselves, especially because they often
possess strong sexual natures and they should be particularly selective about their partners, not putting themselves at
risk. Scorpios need a release or an expressive outlet for their
intense passionate and sexual nature. Channelling their energy productively into creative endeavours or energetically
into sporting pursuits can be useful. Other Scorpios are motivated to join a cause, to champion the underprivileged, or
to defend the underdog.

With their ardent emotions, Scorpios can feel slighted
when they have been hurt. They may have strong personalities but this does not prevent them from falling into the
trap of victim consciousness when they hold on to hurts in
the form of guilt, resentment and bitterness. If these types
of feeling are stored up rather than released, the energy may
have the potential to manifest as problems in their vulnerable areas.

HEALING AND SELF-
DEVELOPMENT FOR SCORPIOS

The mind

If you are a Scorpio, your strong feelings need an outlet and
should not be repressed or stored away. Emotions you carry,
such as hate or vindictiveness, can concentrate and fester
internally. They may manifest negatively from a health point
of view. If you are able to obtain some degree of self-mastery
over your powerful emotions, then these destructive feelings

can be released. In most cases, hanging on to negative emotions only brings suffering to yourself.

Scorpio is ruled by two planets: passionate and energetic Mars, and also Pluto, God of the underworld, said to link with your deep nature and tendency to look beneath the surface of things, even down into the darkness. Pluto is also the planet of transformation, and this concept of change and regeneration can be a potent factor in your life. You instinctively know those times when it is appropriate to root out any aspects of yourself that are no longer useful and replace them with something more positive. To this end, you may encounter periods in life which force a complete upheaval, followed by a healing and reorientation of your living and thinking. You possess enormous power to transform and heal yourself and others if you are willing to let go of old feelings and surrender any need to control. However, your secretiveness and defensiveness can inhibit your own ability to heal as you may find it difficult to allow others to help you.

The body

☛ *Read the Taurus chapter too—your opposite sign*

As Scorpio is a water sign, you respond well to all water sports or therapies where the healing and soothing quality of water is restorative. Since elimination can be one of your vulnerable areas, it is crucial you have a diet sufficient in fluids, minerals, vitamins and fibre. Therapies involving colonic irrigation may appeal to some Scorpios. Past-life regression is one therapy that may be popular, as is rebirthing.

The intensity of your emotions can be a powerful driving force, providing not only physical strength but also great determination and endurance. The more your energy can be channelled constructively and positively into something deeply absorbing, the better for your fulfilment and sense of wellbeing. Others are often drawn to your magnetic personality, as you possess a penetrating energy which, when used to its highest potential, can be directed into a powerful source of healing or benefit for others.

The spirit

USING YOUR INNER POWER AND FINDING YOUR SPIRITUAL MISSION

At certain times we all act like puppets, at the mercy of our emotions. Such behaviour can deprive us of our power and rob us of our peace of mind. This is particularly apt for Scorpio, who is often learning lessons about control of their intense emotions and use of their powerful natures. Once you recognize how emotion can dominate and destroy your peace of mind, you can set about overcoming strong emotions, mastering and training them to work positively for you and, where appropriate, for the good of others. This is not easy for Scorpios who have psyches with deep recesses to purge and demons to defeat, in order to release any lower aspects of their personalities.

☛ For the Soul-lessons, see pp. 13 & 25

Scorpio's soul-lesson is to find inner peace, and to this end life may bring you tests that include opportunities to conquer your strong feelings. By rising above them, you can direct emotional force towards more productive ends. Your ultimate victory comes from shining a light on darkness and confronting and releasing any destructiveness. You will be manifesting your inner power and functioning at your highest potential when you are not ruled and controlled by your passionate emotions, however painful or traumatic they may be. Part of your lesson of learning peace is to release your hold on power over others and learn to use your own power more effectively.

SUGGESTED ESSENCES FOR SCORPIOS

Resolving possible personality imbalances

Rather than deny intense feelings, which can manifest as imbalances in the body, it is in your best interests to learn to come to terms with your deep emotions and integrate them positively into your personality. Your penetrating nature, combined with the courage to look within yourself, means you can confront, clear away and transform any hidden, negative aspects of your psyche. By learning to integrate and transmute these powerful emotions into more constructive channels, you can create peace of mind ultimately.

Coping with intense emotions

With a soul-lesson of inner peace, you are learning to elevate yourself above deep passions and feelings in order to provide a sense of stillness, calm and peace into your life.

Facing up to feelings....

A help in recognizing and handling these intense emotions, powerful moods and strong reactions is the essence *Scarlet Monkeyflower.* It helps you to face up to and deal with any issues involving the use of power, repressed feelings and anger. 'The *Scarlet Monkeyflower* treats a particular state of fear within the human soul: the soul's fear of its own "shadow self" or lower emotions. Those who need this remedy often keep a "lid" on unpleasant emotions' (Kaminski and Katz).

Dealing with emotions....

Providing a strong sense of identity, the gem essence *Tiger's Eye* enables you to deal with strong emotions more easily and not to take things so personally. Helping you discern between your true self and your feelings, this essence enables you to distance your own emotions from the emotions of others.

Transforming feelings....

The transformation of uneasy feelings into love, patience, respect and consideration is a key attribute of *Grape* essence. By helping to change any uncomfortable feelings or negative emotions, this essence brings about a more peaceful and loving nature. Instead of your closing down or shutting yourself off, it helps you to find love within. As you do so, feelings of vulnerability, neediness and other unloving attitudes are released.

Transmuting emotions....

Your strong emotions can evoke fiery feelings ranging from distrust and suspicion to anger, hate and revenge. *Holly* essence helps transmutes these emotions, replacing them with an inner harmony and a loving, tolerant and generous nature.

Holly embodies the principle of love and enables you to open your heart to this energy and radiate it out to others.

> *'I acknowledge my feelings and channel them positively'*

Freeing up fixed and stubborn minds

Your Scorpio mind is curious, deep and piercing, but you can have the tendency to think the worst about things, which is not helpful. As a fixed sign, you can be immovable and set in your ways; no amount of persuasion will change your mind and this can even be to the extent of using your stubbornness to control others.

Uncompromising natures....

The essence of **Fig** helps you, if you have an uncompromising nature, to become more adaptable and openminded. The relaxing energy of this essence frees up self-restraining patterns, transforming them with feelings of self-acceptance, easiness and comfort with oneself.

Detrimental thinking....

Excellent at shifting attachment to patterns that are detrimental to wellbeing, the essence **Stonecrop** breaks through such an attitude. It moves you on when stuck, resistant or stubbornly clinging to the past. Assisting you make transitions in your behaviour, this essence accepts no resistance and enables personal transformations to take place.

Limiting patterns....

The essence **Camellia** eliminates old feelings and self-limiting thought-patterns that you can hold with regard to yourself. Penetrating the self-protective armour that you can sometimes erect, **Camellia** essence inspires shifts in self-attitude. It opens you to your true self: old behaviour patterns make way for flexibility and openness with this essence.

Inflexibility....

According to Sabina Pettitt, the challenges that **Pink Seaweed** essence addresses are 'change and inflexibility'. It can help you to feel comfortable enough to release the past, make way for change and embrace the new. Her affirmation for this essence is: 'I am grounded and secure. I move in the flow of life'.

Set views....

Isopogon essence aids those Scorpios who think they know best for others, or when they refuse to contemplate another's

174 · CENTAURY FOR VIRGO, ROCK ROSE FOR PISCES

viewpoint. It releases the tendency to be bossy or controlling, and facilitates flexibility and understanding if you are one of those people who can be fixed in their views, especially when they think that they are right.

> 'I am comfortable in myself and I
> approach life with flexibility'

Dealing with self-destructive behaviour

A Scorpio with a vindictive side or a tendency to punish others can end up creating barriers and cutting itself off from other people. This self-destructive type can sting itself to death, or 'cut off its nose to spite its face' just as easily as it does this to others.

Releasing repressed emotions....

The following affirmation embodies the forgiving qualities of **Rowan**. 'I experience forgiveness of myself and others and surrender to unconditional, healing love' (Marion Leigh) In shifting detrimental behaviour-patterns, this essence releases deeply-repressed emotions and assists you to give unconditional love, let go of deep hurts and forgive yourself and others.

Open the heart....

For when you are weighed down by strong emotions, *Grass of Parnassus* essence embodies serenity in the face of vulnerability, hurt and sadness. Helping to remove any self-erected protective barriers, its healing qualities uplift the spirit and open the heart to love and peace.

Inner resources....

Sabina Pettitt writes that *Forsythia* essence 'provides motivation towards transformation of old, useless patterns of behaviour—e.g. habits, addictions, thoughts; helps to break addictions'. Whether this is addiction to negative or obsessive ways of thinking, dysfunctional emotion patterns or to actual damaging habits, then *Forsythia* can provide the inner resources and energy required to stimulate change.

Self-acceptance....

The healing ability of **Alpine Azalea** essence increases self-acceptance and brings a strong energy of love into your being. When you are blocked from feeling love for yourself or for another, this essence discharges these imbalances. It helps you to draw upon this love as a strong healing energy for yourself and for others.

Negativity.... If you are a negative Scorpio, you can become stuck in resentment and hostility, often refusing to see how this destructive attitude affects your circumstances. The positive energy of **Willow** essence increases awareness of how your thinking affects the outcome of situations in your life. This essence encourages optimism and hopefulness, so you can take responsibility and constructive steps to be in charge of your life instead of complaining, blaming others or giving up and withdrawing.

> *'I release all destructive behaviour and replace this with love for myself and others'*

Tackling the dark side

The concept of Pluto, one of your ruling planets, is renewal, rebirth, regeneration and transformation. If you are prepared to do some inner personal work, you have the ability to integrate these qualities constructively into your life. You possess the determination and power to instigate moving on and letting go, transforming your vulnerabilities and negativities into strengths. Flushing out Pluto's darkness and bringing in the light, some specially potent remedies of the flower essence world can assist!

Confront.... **Iona Pennywort** essence appears to be made for the individual with issues to confront. Helping you to recognize your shadow self, this essence brings light to thoughts, fears, states of mind and emotions that are negative, distorted or denied. Encouraging you to eke out your hidden side—any unrecognized dark or suspicious thoughts, any hidden remorse or shame—this essence sweeps clean all corners of the psyche. **Iona Pennywort** helps you to face up to, acknowledge and integrate all aspects of yourself.

Illuminate.... **Letting Go** (Hyacinthus 'White Pearl') is an essence for transformation. Its effect is to encourage you to expand your sense of being, so you can release fears or restricting beliefs of yourself or life. The saying for this essence, according to Rose

Titchiner, is, 'Leap, and the net will appear'. This illuminating essence encourages you to move forward into a lighter space of being without old limiting patterns.

Regenerate....   **Snowdrop** (F) essence resonates well with the concept of regeneration, releasing the old and welcoming the new. Any of your dark, destructive and negative traits give way to optimism and hope for the future, with this essence. Releasing the muck of the past, this essence brings in the light necessary for renewal.

Rejuvenate....   The key words for **Menzies Banksia** essence are 'To Live Again'. Vasudeva and Kadambii Barnao write: 'This essence encourages regeneration, renewal and courage, using painful experiences as an opportunity for greater depth and a source of determination to move forward'. When you are blocked in pessimism and fear as a result of past hurts, this healing essence frees up those perceptions and enables you to see beyond them. It introduces a rejuvenating energy, enabling you to embrace life with happiness and hopefulness.

> *'I cleanse any negativity and darkness from
> my being and move forward into the light'*

Submit to a higher power

If you are fearful of the unknown, then this—together with your strong survival techniques and stubbornness—can create barriers, as you can obstinately block anything that does not fit within your framework of the world.

Acceptance....   **Revelation** essence, a combination of Findhorn essences (**Stonecrop, Snowdrop, Holy Thorn** and **Hazel**), increases acceptance of insights and perceptions that are outside our usual understanding. The freedom and detachment that this essence brings enables you to move forward with vitality and deeper wisdom, relinquishing self-imposed limitations.

Surrender....   If you are a Scorpio that is too ego-invested, then it is more difficult for you to change, grow and develop. **Round-Leaved Sundew** essence releases attachments at this level. Steve Johnson writes, 'the ego is a part of the human being that is necessary for survival in this dimension. Our task is not to diminish the ego, but rather to give it appropriate acknowledgment and support. This essence teaches us how to bring the strength and tenacity of the ego into harmony and balance with the wisdom and guidance of the higher self'. It brings you the willingness to surrender to higher knowledge in order to develop and progress.

Higher aspirations....

The keywords for **Apple** (F) essence are 'higher purpose and will-to-good' (Marion Leigh). Uniting your desires with your higher aspirations, **Apple** helps you to become conscious of how to realign any lower aspects of your nature to serve better ends. It helps you to realize how to develop and channel your energies productively and for the best.

> *'I move away from self-imposed limits
> and open to higher wisdom'*

Balancing Scorpio energy

Highly sensitive to others, you need to be cocooned against any influences that leave you vulnerable and unbalanced. Choosing your company wisely and seeing life positively is helpful to your wellbeing. By accepting certain situations, releasing grudges, healing past hurts and rising above any unhappiness, you can use your regenerative powers to go forward, renewed and revitalized.

Protection from the energies of others

So good are you at picking up another's feelings and moods, that you can usually sense what another feels, or the dynamics of a situation, without having had a verbal explanation.

Shielding....

If you easily take on the feelings or absorb the energies of others, you may benefit from **Fringed Violet** essence. The qualities of this essence provide protection from the negative and draining energies of other people. Helping to keep your life-force intact and balanced, this essence can also be taken after shock, trauma or surgery.

Resilience....

The shielding strength of **Hybrid Pink Fairy Cowslip Orchid** essence creates a wellbeing note of inner strength and resilience. You become less affected by the emotions of others and are able to respond sensitively rather than reacting emotionally with this essence.

Defending.... **Guardian** is a combination of several Alaskan essences and extremely useful for all sensitive people. It protects by surrounding you with a strong energetic boundary, preventing the absorption of unwanted energies. Defended and protected, you can feel safe and guarded in your own space with the help of this essence.

Protecting.... Not only protecting on an outer level, the essence of **Yellow Yarrow** allows you to soften inwardly. This is appropriate if you create barriers and close down emotionally when feeling defenceless and vulnerable.

> *'I am totally protected and remain*
> *unaffected by inharmonious energies'*

Freeing up bitterness

A wronged Scorpio does not usually forget, and will either settle a score or wait a long time to get even, often holding lingering bitterness in their body. Not a wise choice, this may result in emotional 'dis-ease' or physical illness.

Forgiveness.... Clearing away hatred, anger and blocked feelings, **Mountain Devil** essence infuses feelings of forgiveness, acceptance and unconditional love. Referring to those who need this essence, Ian White (ABFE) writes that 'as these people are poisoning themselves with hatred and resentment, they may develop illnesses'. This essence tackles revengeful, suspicious, jealous and envious states (which reflect a lack of self-love), by instilling goodwill and compassionate feelings toward yourself and others.

Resentment.... The actual physical characteristics of a flower can represent its healing abilities. Not surprisingly, the healing attributes of the spiky shrub **Dagger Hakea** bring forgiveness to those individuals who are prickly in their interactions with others. Freeing up bitterness and grudges, this essence opens up your feelings, instilling lightness and increasing vitality. It enables antipathy, aggression or stored-away anger to give way to kindness.

SCORPIO (OCTOBER 24–NOVEMBER 22) · 179

Negativity....

The saying for **Cape Bluebell** essence is 'Freeing the Past' (Barnao), which describes this essence's renewing qualities. Allowing a release of negativity, pain and bitterness, it heals your feelings of resentment, jealousy or blame, inspiring acceptance in others and a joy of life.

Release of judgment....

The forgiving energy of **Phoenix Rebirth** essence makes it possible to release judgments of yourself and others and to forgive on a deep level. Vengeance, anger and reprisal give way to understanding and compassion with this essence. It frees up your perception of yourself as a victim—after all, what use is it, if we hold on to the image of ourselves as the injured party?

> *'I have only understanding, compassion and forgiveness for myself and others'*

Healing deep wounds and hurts

Moving on from hurts and anguish will release the energy invested in issues where there is held pain, and allow it to be redirected positively.

Understanding....

Blue Elf Viola essence helps you get in touch with any deep-seated anger and frustration. The following affirmation, according to Steve Johnson, expresses this essence's ability to understand and deal calmly with the issues that originally contributed to these feelings. 'I understand the seeds of my anger and release them into love. What I feel, I can heal'.

Objectivity....

Imbuing compassion, peace and serenity for yourself and others, **Green Bog Orchid** essence supports the healing of issues and blockages held in the heart. As it confronts deeply-held concerns, this essence enables you to embrace them with objectivity. In addition to expanding your self-understanding, it provides a deeper awareness of nature.

Trust....

If you are defensive or suspicious of another's motives, it may make you reluctant to reveal yourself. This, coupled with your deep need for privacy, can tend to make you a loner. Moreover, sometimes slipping into negative patterns to protect yourself can sabotage your health and happiness. The essence **Pink Mulla Mulla** guards you from being hurt or taken advantage of by others and breaks through this resistance. Healing deep wounds in the psyche, it instils trust and diminishes the fear of revealing yourself to others.

Freeing....   If you find yourself in a constant state of discontent, you can be fearful of looking too deeply into yourself. Alternatively, you can feel blocked and restricted by events that have occurred in your past. The essence of **Sitka Burnet** destroys these fears, providing awareness of the real issues to be addressed, not the emotions attached to them. The freeing energy of this essence allows you to recognize the lessons attached to these issues and to release them and move on.

> *'All painful wounds in my psyche are healed
> and all distressing emotions are cleared'*

Moderating highly-sensitive capabilities

In keeping with the subjects of other water signs, Scorpios are very intuitive and perceptive. This makes you highly receptive to events or sensations that are beyond your normal senses, something which in turn may leave you feeling very vulnerable and cause you to worry unnecessarily.

Trepidation....   If you are frightened by any aspect of the occult, the supporting essence **Purple Monkeyflower** instils calm. It establishes a love-based approach to spirituality, so you feel safe to be guided and trusting in your own spirituality, instead of feeling alarm or trepidation around these matters.

Overwhelmed....   The essence of **Lavender** is for those people who are too absorbent psychically. It establishes an emotional balance so that you do not become overwrought with subtle influences that can deplete energy, create disturbances on a physical level and produce nervous problems. It moderates and refines your spiritual capabilities so they are not out of step or overwhelming your physical body.

Fear....   **Bush Iris** essence provides a safe awareness of spirituality at the same time as eliminating fears of your psychic abilities.

Resistance....   If you feel unable to share your perceptions with others or to make sense of them in a practical way, then **Northern**

Twayblade essence enables you to find a way of combining and grounding spiritual aspects into physical life. It removes fears and resistance so you do not doubt what you experience or see, enabling you to easily share these insights with others.

> '*I am calm and comfortable with my insights and perceptions*'

Relating and communicating

Although adept at understanding others, you hate feeling vulnerable and like to be in charge. The more manipulative Scorpio may resort to manipulating others or using control to keep those they care about in a state of attachment. Those who fear dependence can be critical and possessive of loved ones, gaining affection by force. Your capacity to understand how another feels and to be able to regenerate and revitalize them is a positive use of your characteristics.

Loving without expectations

Although fiercely loyal and protective, when out of balance you can be too demanding or too attached to loved ones.

Selfless love....

Chicory essence promotes a feeling of safety and security. Shifting self-centredness, it enables you to give love and devotion to others selflessly, without conditions or expectations. It fills up and satisfies that fearful, bottomless-pit feeling with an endless supply of self-love. Demanding behaviour and need for attention are changed into positive feelings of warmth and care for others with this essence.

Self-fulfilment....

The self-appreciation and inner contentment that *Snakebush* essence imparts, enables needy Scorpios to release this pattern. Teaching wisdom in loving, this essence provides self-fulfilment, so that you do not love others from a perspective of needing to be loved, and do not give love to others when it is not appreciated. Healing feelings of bitterness and inspiring the independence of mind to move from submissive relationships, *Snakebush* helps create healthy ones.

Unconditional Love....	**Bleeding Heart** essence fosters the energy of unconditional love, so that your relationships are not based on possessiveness or dependence. It inspires independence in relationships, in addition to providing support at times of broken-heartedness.
Positivity....	If you are coping with emotional traumas and relationship break-ups, the assistance of **Black Kangaroo Paw** essence heals hurt, hatred, resentment and angry feelings. It inspires you to go forward in life, leaving pain behind. The meditation poem for this essence says this nicely: 'I am part of all Life I watching it and within it also. I Buffeted by storms I I do not lose my way. I I keep my eyes on the Light I and fly freely to joy' (Barnao).
Sincerity....	**Pale Sundew** essence purifies the heart, awakening your consciousness to any controlling or manipulative behaviour you may be showing, and the effect this has on others. It awakens those parts of your psyche that need light and reveals awareness of your actions. Deceptive tactics, shallow feelings or insincere deeds are exposed, transformed and replaced by sincerity and genuineness with this essence.

> *'I love unconditionally and selflessly'*

Enhancing compassion and tolerance

Although sensitive and caring, you can sometimes be inflexible, especially when hurt or fearful. The following essences enhance understanding and consideration for others.

Tolerance....	In addition to removing rigidity and resistance to change, **Bauhinia** essence increases flexibility and tolerance. Any attitudes of opposition and unwillingness can now give way to a more agreeable and adaptable manner, wherein you become less narrow-minded and more accepting of people and situations.
Abundance....	Assisting you to look within, **Bluebell** (AB) essence helps open the heart to the concept of love and abundance. If you feel cut off from your emotions, this essence enables you to let go of fear and encourages loving and giving.
Consider-ation....	Increasing your tolerance and sensitivity, **Beech** essence transforms any limited, restrictive belief-patterns and judgments

you may hold about others. The strongly defensive Scorpio with narrow views can be a law unto him- or herself! **Beech** essence opens this type up to a higher aspect of themselves, thus reducing inner rigidity and encouraging easiness, sympathy and consideration for others.

Willingness.... The flower essence **Slender Rice Flower** inspires acceptance and harmony. Promoting flexibility and the willingness to listen to others, it increases your ability to develop understanding and humility in relationships.

Nurturing.... **Peach** essence, 'The Selfless Mother' (Lila Devi), embodies supportive and caring qualities. It boosts concern and nurturing for others when you need to put another's needs before your own.

Empathy.... Imparting awareness of others, the essence of **Yellow Star Tulip** replaces insensitivity with empathy, consideration and receptivity. It heightens awareness of how your own actions affect others, in addition to enhancing sensitivity, compassion and caring for others.

> *'I possess great understanding,*
> *consideration and compassion for others'*

The Scorpio sting

Despite keeping most of your true nature concealed beneath the surface, your sensitive character may incline you to react moodily, touchily or with irritation towards others at times.

Purifying.... Lila Devi calls **Blackberry** essence the 'All-Purpose Purifier'. It cleanses unkindness, sharp words, sarcasm and insults from your psyche, and raises your vibration so thoughts and words are exchanged with the awareness of how they affect others.

Lessening overreaction.... Another fruit essence, **Raspberry,** calms touchy natures that tend to react intensely to situations, especially when clouded by emotions. It helps transform any harmful or negative emotions, replacing insensitivity with wisdom, increased understanding and benevolence for others. Overreaction lessens with this essence, so the Scorpio who tends to blame others takes responsibility for his or her feelings and responses.

Opening up....   **Pink Mulla Mulla** essence is for spiteful words. When you have suffered hurts, or are suspicious and guarded of the motives of others, you may have protected yourself from further hurt by using unkindness or words to keep people at a safe distance. Fear of being hurt can prompt you to use words as a form of defence; your words often bear no resemblance to what you actually feel. This essence works with deep levels of resistance, inspiring trust and opening you up to interact freely with others.

Respon-sibility....   Feelings of resentment, revenge and vindictiveness are released with **Donkey Orchid** essence. Instilling feelings of detachment and peace, this essence assists you to walk away from blame, resentment and unforgiveness. It helps you to be responsible for your actions and reactions in life and not to hang on to painful issues that may cause you pain.

Detachment....   If you are easily aggravated by others, **Orange Spiked Pea** essence brings a healing detachment, enabling you to express yourself in a calm manner without exploding in self-defence. It is known as 'The Articulation of Expression'. According to Vasudeva and Kadambii Barnao, 'the healing helps one to articulate feelings in a positive way and be able to walk away from a verbal fight when the only purpose from the other person is to inflict a sense of inferiority or shame. One then learns the beauty of detachment and mastery of the Self'. These are important words for a Scorpio, who can be mortified at the thought of not having the upper hand or losing his or her dignity.

A safe place....   The essence of *Achillea Millefolium*, known as **Peaceful Detachment**, creates objectivity if you find yourself getting dragged into an issue or reacting from either a fearful or ego perspective. This essence enables you to be in a safe place in relation to others; above the need to react and protected from oversensitivity.

> *'I respond peacefully and express myself with calm detachment'*

The right use of power

Increasing your sense of inner authority and resolving imbalances of power, the following essences help you to interact wisely with others.

SCORPIO (OCTOBER 24–NOVEMBER 22) · 185

Wise authority....	The essence of *Crocus Thomasinianus* 'Royal', known as **True Power**, helps resolve issues around the abuse of power, such as controlling and manipulative behaviour. Reminding us all that true power comes from within not from unhealthy struggles on an external level, this essence enables you to become centred in your own wise authority. The feeling of love and compassion this essence instils heals the need for outer recognition and approval and helps you relate with sensitivity and thoughtfulness.
Reconnecting with the power of love....	Introducing a consciousness of compassion and sensitivity, the essence **Rough Bluebell** is for the thoughtless or hurtful Scorpio, particularly when they are centred in achieving their own needs. **Rough Bluebell** essence assists you in eliminating any abusive or exploitative ways of relating. Instilling the right use of your power, creating kindness and concern for the needs of others, it reconnects you with the power of love.
Positive authority....	**Rose Alba** is the essence for individual power and strength. Marion Leigh writes the following with regard to the qualities that can be strengthened by **Rose Alba**. 'Without love, power can be misused. Through learned control-patterns and feelings of inadequacy or pride, the lower self or ego can undermine the inner authority or the True Self'. This essence addresses inappropriate, overbearing expressions of power and control. By increasing your emotional security and inner authority, it enables a positive expression of an individual's personal power.
Powerless-ness....	When experiencing emotional turmoil, you can feel powerless, often reacting intensely in order to protect yourself from what you perceive as external attack. The stabilizing energy of **Broccoli** essence enhances personal power, so that you are able to maintain your balance on all levels, without closing down or scattering your forces. You can then tackle inner emotional issues with strength and as a fully-functioning unit.

'I am balanced and centred in my own authority'

Resolving possible physical imbalances

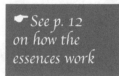

☞ See p. 12 on how the essences work

Please note that throughout this book suggestions of a medical nature are not in any way claiming that the essences will cure disease, and should not be followed as a substitute to consulting a qualified medical practitioner.

Elimination

Since Scorpios have a general tendency to retention, keeping hold of your feelings can result in constipation. The nurturing, soft energy of *Barnacle* essence heals bowel dysfunctions. When you are stubborn and resistant, its gentle energy gets things flowing. *Starfish* essence is for release on all levels. Assisting you in times of grief, it also carries away old attachments and eliminates impurities from the body, mind or spirit. A third essence, *Pink Seaweed*, is also used for constipation, in addition to freeing up the past, encouraging flexibility and relieving resistance to change.

Helpful in dissolving rigid feelings, *Poison Hemlock* essence enables things to 'get going and keep moving'. This essence works both on a mental and physical level. Sabina Pettitt writes: 'Physically it acts on holding patterns in the body—constipation, fluid retention, overweight and any kind of paralysis in the physical structure of the nervous system'. Working on any aspect of elimination and stuckness, the essence of *Camellia* moves old energy forward into new thoughts and new ways of being.

Reproductive area

The challenge of *Sea Lettuce* essence is in 'facing the dark side'. Healing the shadow, this is an essence of purification and release and 'can be used when healing is required for the reproductive organs or the bowels' (Sabina Pettitt). Its soothing energy brings relief for inflammatory conditions in these areas. Scorpio rules the sexual and reproductive organs, which can also be vulnerable areas for their opposite sign, Taurus. *She Oak* essence helps with menstrual and female reproductive problems and *Macrozamia* essence can be used for imbalances and blockages related to both the female and male sexual organs and their functions. Two other essences that work on both male and female reproductive issues are *Watermelon* and *Pomegranate*.

The Bladder

Debbie Shapiro writes that the 'urinary tract is where we let go of our negative feelings, maintaining a balance in our system by doing so. Any inflammation implies a build-up of anger, resentment, irritation or other 'hot' feelings. This indicates we have an excess of negative emotions to the point where the urinary system is unable to deal with them in the normal way'. As the essence *Dagger Hakea* frees up feelings of bitterness, anger or resentment in the psyche, it also releases this negative energy from being held in the bladder area. *Mountain Devil* essence imparts feelings of forgiveness, avoiding the poison of hatred and resentment that may develop into discomfort in this area.

Brown Kelp essence affects the bladder and is helpful in controlling the storage of water and maintaining adequate reservoirs of bodily fluids. Also helping to provide sufficient fluid balance, *Sponge* essence is for letting go and for filtering impurities from one's mind. Judy Griffin (FTH) writes that '*Begonia* allows one to feel more trusting and secure in life'. This is important, in that she links feeling tense and threatened by life with the bladder. She continues that 'holding tension within oneself may affect the bladder by causing cramping or by withholding fluids. Bladder infections may occur'.

9. THE SAGITTARIUS OUTLOOK ON LIFE AND HEALTH

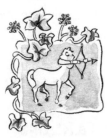

Sagittarius

November 22–
December 22

Quality & element:
Mutable Fire

Ruler: Jupiter

Opposite sign:
Gemini

Soul-lesson: Love

CONSTITUTION

SAGITTARIANS are happiest when they have plenty of change and variety in their lives. Being cooped up indoors is not usually for them; they can feel restricted and restless. Activity, outdoor life and freedom of movement are usually essential elements they need to build into their lives. Generally, this is not difficult as the typical Sagittarian is either sporty or motivated to pursue an energetic lifestyle of some sort. Sagittarians also require a fair amount of intellectual stimulation and can make excellent students. Their directness, together with a concern for truth, honesty and justice usually means they say exactly what is on their minds. With generous spirits and great enthusiasm, their cheerful, optimistic view of life and their ability to change negatives into positives ensure they are well-liked by others.

Implications for health

Jupiter, Sagittarius's ruling planet, rules the liver, the largest organ in the body, whose function is to convert and store nutrients for the body. Jupiter is the largest planet in our solar system, and not surprisingly its size is echoed in the Sagittarian approach to life. Expansive by nature, Sagittarians like to do things in a big way—but in some of them this can result in excess and indulgence. The liver is often the area of their bodies to suffer, so therefore it is important that they moderate their intake of rich foods and the consumption of alcohol.

In keeping with this principle of expansion, Sagittarians can scatter their energies. Initiating many things at once, they can find themselves taking on more than they can manage, and leaving much incomplete! The symbol for Sagittarius depicts the archer shooting arrows. Not always sure of their goals or able to see a clear target, Sagittarian people tend to fire themselves forward without much thought, particularly when young. Perhaps it is their very love of adventure that makes them impulsive. Their reckless approach to life sometimes causes accidents or mishaps, while their tendency to take risks can result in them getting into scrapes.

HEALING AND SELF-DEVELOPMENT FOR SAGITTARIANS

The mind

If you are a Sagittarian, you are likely to be concerned with expansion, movement or travel. If for any reason your love of freedom or activity is curtailed or limited physically in some way, through confinements or difficulties that restrict your movements, then this forces you instead to seek mental travel, expansion and freedom of the mind. It is useful that as well as having an active body you are also likely to have an active and inquisitive mind! By reflecting on life, you can open your mind to the mysteries of the universe. In your quest for wisdom you can broaden your thinking through studies such as philosophy, belief-systems or metaphysics. Openminded Sagittarians understand that as they overcome whatever life throws their way, other opportunities will be presented to them to satisfy their energies.

Some Sagittarians can suppress feelings of frustration and anger, and may even resort to alcohol to escape or deny these feelings. If you look to your opposite sign of Gemini, it can be helpful to adopt this sign's healthy quality of outward expression, rather than feeling restricted and holding back your thoughts.

The body

Jupiter's enlarging influence can inappropriately urge Sagittarians to increase their appetites and expand their waistlines! With this in mind, it is to your benefit to take some form of exercise or sporting activity, where exercise of the thighs and buttocks especially will stop you putting on weight in this area. You may be on the sports field often, but your association with horses can often find you at the stables. This energetic way of occupying your time is infinitely more productive than limiting your interest of horses to the racecourse or betting shop (gambling is another Jupiterian preoccupation)!

Sagittarius rules the sciatic nerve, running down the back of the legs. Pain here, according to Debbie Shapiro's THE BODYMIND WORKBOOK, suggests that a sense of duty, or maybe doubt or fear, is connected with the direction you are taking in life. If you have trouble in the sciatic nerve—or anywhere in the hips, buttocks, lumbar or pelvic area—it may be that you bury or sit on something that you are not wanting to face up to. You may be hiding something that you do not want others to see or know about. Debbie Shapiro goes on to say that the pelvis is our area of relationship and communication, and can have a lot to do with fears and conflicts to do with our security, our loved ones, family or friends.

☞ Read the Gemini chapter too—your opposite sign.

The spirit

USING YOUR INNER POWER AND FINDING YOUR SPIRITUAL MISSION

Consistent with your restlessness and love of movement, you enjoy being here, there and everywhere, sometimes firing your (metaphorical) arrows indiscriminately in a quest to find your direction and place in life. Your true inner power, though, comes from being able calmly to direct this random energy, to still the body and mind and to seek and develop true wisdom and intuition.

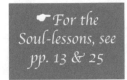

☞ For the Soul-lessons, see pp. 13 & 25

Along with all fire-sign people, your soul-lesson is love. For Sagittarius, especially, this implies love of a greater wisdom or knowledge, in addition to love for others or self-love. Sagittarians are learning about consistency, which often involves relationships, especially with those they love. The wise Sagittarian searches for truth so that they can stand as a sage: one with wisdom and knowledge to whom others come for advice and inspiration.

SUGGESTED ESSENCES FOR SAGITTARIANS

Resolving possible personality imbalances

You can be the life and soul of the party—carefree, outgoing and optimistic on an outer level—but this behaviour can disguise inner mental anguish and a difficulty in expressing your fears. You prefer to be free, to move around ready for the next adventure in life without too many ties or responsibilities. This approach can take you on many journeys, some physically and some internally, as the spiritual seeker.

Releasing suppressed feelings

When agitated and worried, you can put on a brave face and smile through adversities. Not discussing your inner worries with anyone, you dislike others to see you as other than positive, or in any way vulnerable. Neither do you find it easy to integrate any negative experiences you have in life or the less positive aspects of your personality. Some Sagittarians may resort to drinks and drugs to calm their anxieties.

Taking the self lightly....	**Agrimony** essence enables you to communicate your worries more easily to others and to take yourself more lightly. This essence makes it easier for you to recognize, integrate and accept all parts of yourself. Providing you with the inner strength and calmness to see your problems and worries from a higher perspective, it also encourages you in your search for peace within.
Freeing up the emotions....	Assisting you more easily to share your feelings with others, the essence **Bluebell** (AB) opens the heart, enabling suppressed or denied feelings to be voiced. Infusing your being with feelings of joy and happiness, this essence helps free up closed, rigid and unexpressed emotions.
Expressing strong emotions....	The affirmation for **Meadow Sage** essence, according to Judy Griffin, is 'I choose my words wisely'. Helping you to express strong emotions such as anger without guilt or spite, this essence permits a healthy expression of balanced emotions.
Releasing tension....	Another essence in Judy Griffin's 'Petite Fleur' collection, particularly for the suppression of anger, is **Pink Geranium**. She writes (FTH) that this essence 'will ease the emotional pain and enable the personality to laugh and enjoy life again. The individual will become aware of who (or what) is causing anger and take steps to rectify the situation. They will learn to constructively release tension and anger without transferring anger to others'.

> *'I am free to express my feelings'*

Being comfortable with responsibility

The freedom-loving Sagittarian can be reluctant to accept responsibility. The following essences help to instil this quality.

Dependable....	**Many-Headed Dryandra** essence brings one the maturity necessary to commit to others, or to any area of life that requires consistency or dedication. This essence unites fulfilment with consistent commitment, encouraging you to find pleasure from being stable and dependable in life.

SAGITTARIUS (NOVEMBER 22–DECEMBER 22) · 193

Respon-
sibility....

Integrating responsibility with your desires, the selfless energy of **Christmas Tree-Kanya** essence is right for the inconsistent, unreliable or self-absorbed Sagittarian. This essence reorientates self-centred desires, along with restlessness and non-accountable behaviour, by introducing a consciousness of caring. It helps you to feel far more content and satisfied with being answerable to another or sharing responsibilities with others.

Consistency....

Fear and avoidance of responsibility can also be addressed by **Illawarra Flame Tree** essence. If you find it hard to use your potential because you are overwhelmed by the consistency and commitment required to develop it, this essence brings strength and self-reliance.

Satisfaction....

Appropriate for the typical Sagittarian psyche, **Red Beak Orchid** essence unites responsibility with desire. It is useful if your unfulfilled desires create frustration and anger. According to Vasudeva and Kadambii Barnao, the purpose of this essence is 'to resolve the internal conflict between desire and duties, personal expression and responsibilities'. The healing energies of this essence also help to set various desires in one major direction, so an individual can become more satisfied and resolute.

> *'I am responsible, dependable and consistent'*

In the pursuit of inner wisdom

You are the explorer and the adventurer. If, in your quest for wisdom and truth, you cannot journey far afield physically, you can venture inwardly in pursuit of knowledge.

Deepening
awareness....

By exploring your unconscious mind, you can deepen your awareness and tap into unlimited knowledge. **Lady's Mantle** essence takes you on this journey, especially if you are over-rational or easily distracted. It inspires you to look within and trust your wise inner knowing.

Intuition....

Keeping you in tune with your gut feelings, **Bush Fuchsia** essence enhances intuition and increases your trust in being guided and following these inner observations. This essence also brings confidence and clarity to speak or teach with conviction.

Trust.... You make a good teacher, but you can also benefit by accessing your own inner teacher. Helping you contact your own source of wisdom, *Scots Pine* essence helps you find truths and answers. The affirmation for this essence, by Marion Leigh, is 'I am receptive to the truth and wisdom within my being'. It enables you to trust in your inner direction, insights and perceptions.

Clarity.... As a thought-amplifier, *Sapphire* gem essence acts on the intellect, bringing inspiration and clarity to your thinking. If you feel you are reaching towards higher realms for mental travel, *Sapphire* motivates and assists you in your search for spiritual enlightenment. It also helps focus your responsibility and concentrate your purpose in life.

> 'Knowledge brings me wisdom and satisfaction'

Manifesting your goals

If you are a typically passionate and enthusiastic Sagittarian, then your energy needs a direction. However, with your desire to experience as much as possible, you can sometimes launch into indiscriminate behaviour or impractical activities. It is characteristic of the Sagittarian to leap into something without thinking or planning a particular outcome.

Facing up to consequences.... *Wattle* essence has a mature energy that ensures you become aware of reality and face up to situations. The wisdom of this essence encourages you to understand the consequences of your actions and to discern good judgment in all your choices.

The right choice.... Assisting Sagittarians with various options, *Pippsissewa* essence helps you to make the right decision or to select the correct path in life. According to Sabina Pettitt, this essence also 'helps resolve the frustration around having made a choice which seems not to turn out the way we thought it would. Instead of wasting energy bewailing where we find ourselves, the essence will help move us to the point of power in the present where we can make a new choice'.

Endurance.... When things get tough and require dedication to go on, some Sagittarians would rather opt out. *Silver Princess* essence inspires endurance and determination in these circumstances. Rather than you feeling frustrated or admitting defeat, it encourages your inner strength to keep going, to overcome obstacles and to tackle difficulties. It points to new avenues at times of frustration or when things appear stagnant or at a dead end.

Direction....

To help you to get in touch with the work you born to do, **Sapphire** gem essence brings you clarity for direction in your life's purpose. In addition to increasing your awareness, **Sapphire** essence also helps you to align spiritual responsibilities with your actual physical capabilities.

Gathering your forces....

The empowering energy of **Laurel** essence enables you to find your own resources to manifest the ideals and ideas that are important to you. It enables you to gather your forces and put them into action. It is useful if you tend to give up easily or procrastinate, or may fail to take a necessary risk. It helps you to choose the opportunities that are in alignment with your highest truth and the commitment to bring forth your potential.

'*I possess the purpose and dedication to achieve my goals*'

Balancing Sagittarian energy

If you are too zealous, overly confident, overly enthusiastic or overly energetic, then burn-out can result. You are best with challenges, goals or projects to focus on, but distractions can result in lost concentration or a tendency to go off on a tangent. If you spread yourself too thinly you become overwhelmed and scattered. Confusion around your opportunities, putting off and postponing activities and objectives, is another thing that can affect your energy.

Misuse of fiery energy

As a Sagittarian it is important for you to broaden your horizons by widening your experiences, but if you are the intense type, you can take the principle of expansion to the extreme or go over the top, which may result in exhaustion.

Over-exuberance....	The essence ***Vervain*** enhances your self-discipline and restraint, lessening your over-exuberant states and any squandering of energy. It also takes in hand the fanatical Sagittarian who is passionate about what they believe and insistent on convincing others of those beliefs.
Recklessness....	Reckless and rash types can benefit from the relaxed energy of ***Kangaroo Paw*** essence. Helping you cope with hasty and careless behaviour, this essence inspires you to retain your high spirits and spontaneity without impetuosity and impulsive behaviour wasting your energy. It also helps you to develop awareness of any time you are putting yourself in jeopardy or taking unnecessary risks.
Impatience....	With ***Impatiens*** essence, you will find that you are calmer and less bothered about hasty activities. Encouraging you to take life at a slower and safer pace, this essence lessens thoughtless and careless actions by increasing restraint and patience.
Over the top....	If you are a Sagittarian with an over-abundance of fiery will, ***Aloe Vera*** essence helps to bring moderation. It makes it easier for you to accomplish your goals without neglecting other aspects of yourself or life. This essence is rejuvenating and renewing at the same time as bringing your inner forces into balanced alignment with the physical.

> *'I use my energy wisely and productively'*

Focus and purpose

Although you are delightfully spontaneous and enthusiastically motivated, your tendency to take on too many projects or interests at the same time can result in you becoming too distracted to complete what you have undertaken.

Con-centration....	When help is needed to consolidate your thoughts and complete a goal, ***Pink Trumpet Flower*** essence can assist you. Particularly good if you tend to skip the details and fail to plan ahead, it encourages you to maintain clarity and purpose in order to realize your objectives. Increasing your inner strength, this essence has the ability to eliminate distractions and to maintain your thinking in a very direct manner. It brings

SAGITTARIUS (NOVEMBER 22–DECEMBER 22) · 197

consistent mental strength, so your mind does not wander or lose its concentration until the job is done.

Continuity.... Eager to experience as much as you can, your flexibility makes it easy for you to adapt to new situations, but your variable nature can make you easily bored. If you undertake too many new commitments or tasks, your energy can become scattered and unproductive. *Peach-Flowered Tea-Tree* essence replaces any tendency to unpredictability or to fluctuate from one extreme to another. This essence instils constancy where inconsistency and boredom existed, facilitating your following projects through rather than losing interest and wasting energy.

Purpose.... The essence of *Sundew* is right for the daydreamy Sagittarian who would prefer to escape and not face up to real life. Feelings of disconnectedness, indecision, procrastination or vagueness are replaced with decisiveness and the awareness of being firmly in the present. Returning you to the here and now, this essence increases concentration and purposefulness if you are unrealistically optimistic or tending to deny reality. It can also be healing if you are inclined to use drugs to avoid reality.

> **'My vision is clear and focused'**

Get on with it!

Along with the subjects of other fire signs, you possess great enthusiasm to start projects but your fidgety nature can mean you lose interest or put things off. Nothing is more draining than when people defer and delay and become locked into patterns of procrastination. If you make excuses, or do not have the strength of will to commit to completing tasks, this can make you frustrated and weary.

Procrastination.... The energizing essence, *Corn*, gets you moving. Increasing vitality and willpower, it positively creates energy and enthusiasm. Replacing sluggishness and lethargy, you can no longer postpone things or drag your feet with this essence. Its energy is initiating and willing, enabling you to commit to getting things done and not putting them off.

Excuses....	Individuals who need *Coconut* essence make excuses or find problems that prevent them completing their objectives. If you are unable to honour commitments or tend to avoid finalizing something, then this essence implants the sustenance and dedication necessary to accomplish your goals. While *Corn* essence provides the motivation for beginning new endeavours, *Coconut* essence instils committed and persevering energy in order to complete efforts.
Indecision....	*Scleranthus* essence assists the Sagittarian who is indecisive and restless, inclined to behaviour that is changeable and unreliable. If you tend to put off or delay matters, this essence restores a sense of balance, increases your determination and providing you with the ability to be decisive and strong-minded.
Self-restriction....	If frustration and restlessness are reasons behind not meeting your goals, *Hazel* essence releases the knots that are tied in the way of realizing your objectives. It is a helpful essence if you impose limitations on yourself, or if fear stands in the way of allowing you to fulfil your intentions. *Hazel* essence frees up any restricting perceptions you may have around your purpose and progress in life. It unites direction and perseverance, together with a trust in the universe that your potential will unfold. This essence creates the contentment to flow with life knowing that your own life is progressing just as it should.
Lack of focus....	The empowering essence *Sticky Geranium* ensures that all levels of your 'being' work together. This essence increases the ability to work as a whole, physically, mentally, emotionally and spiritually, so you can move forward with clarity instead of in an unfocused way or lethargically. It frees up old forgotten levels of programming that can limit and restrict you from reaching your highest potential.

> *'I am committed to achieving my goals'*

Scattered energy

Like many subjects of your opposite sign Gemini, you are happy doing at least two things at once, but if you take on more than you can manage your energy can become diffused and scattered.

Balance....	Restoring a sense of inner balance, *Scleranthus* essence not only helps you act decisively, it also calms changeable, restless and unfocused energy.
Discipline....	In order for you to be able to complete undertakings without getting frustrated and giving up easily, the essence *Wandering Jew* helps produce the necessary discipline and patience. This essence enables you to combine your ideas and reasoned thinking with consistent energy, assisting you to achieve in all your endeavours.
Composure....	Your tendency to scatter your forces often destroys the harmony between the body and the mind, sometimes resulting in nervous exhaustion. The essence *Hops Bush* earths overactive, frenetic energy. It calms these distracted and hectic energies, encouraging you to establish a more composed and healthy pace to life and to be in better step with your entire being.
Focus....	If you are dissipating your energy through rushing around, the antidote for this sort of behaviour is *Jacaranda* essence. This is the correct essence if, rather than mastering one thing well, you end up with several incomplete projects. The positive quality of poise that it instils encourages you to take on only those actions that you can complete successfully. Rather than rushing around madly without actually accomplishing anything, you can maintain a clear head and focus on achieving with this essence.

'My direction is focused'

Keeping the spark alight

Naturally optimistic, you have a fire and passion for life. Your humour is a good tonic not only for yourself but for others too: it is beneficial and healing. When worn down by harsh circumstances or disillusioned because life does not live up to your ideals, however, you can lose this spark and zest.

Joyful expectation....	The lightening up-essence *Sunshine Wattle* alleviates burdensome thinking and helps you to approach life with joyful expectation. Difficult times you may have endured in the past may have created negative and pessimistic beliefs that these hardships continue into the future. *Sunshine Wattle* essence

enables you to perceive life differently and to see the future with optimism. It enables you to go forward with belief in yourself and the faith that things will work out for you.

Simplify issues....

The little flowers of the **Blue Lupin** are shaped like the organ of the liver, which links this essence nicely with Sagittarius on a physical level. On a mental level this essence simplifies issues, releases anger that can be harmful to the liver, and provides clarity so are not confused by a myriad of different ideas. '**Blue Lupin** can help to alleviate feelings of depression which arise from not being able "to see the forest for the trees" and helps us to focus our attention', says Sabina Pettitt.

Lightheartedness....

The essence of **Yellow Flag Flower** helps you to maintain your carefree and jovial manner even when things get tough. The strength of this essence allows you to cope with difficult situations without becoming gloomy and downhearted.

Playfulness....

Sustaining during stressful times, **Zinnia** essence helps you to remain lighthearted, cheerful and humorous. It restores playfulness, joy and humour, if life becomes heavy and serious. 'The message of **Zinnia** is not that one's life should be frivolous or irresponsible, but rather that qualities of playfulness and laughter can be brought to one's work and daily responsibilities' (Kaminski and Katz).

> *'I am glowing with life and positivity'*

Relating and communicating

Cheerful, kind, good-humoured and fun-loving, Sagittarians are usually liked by others. Your presence is inspiring and uplifting, but your tendency to be outspoken or to put your foot in your mouth sometimes means that you can be seen as tactless. Many Sagittarians prefer the flexibility of several uncommitted relationships to being tied down. To avoid feeling trapped, it is preferable that you retain some degree of freedom of movement if you are involved in a relationship.

Handling commitment with others

A typical Sagittarian fears commitment and responsibility because they feel it will curtail their freedom. Instead of pulling away from relationships, strength and dedication are called for. Preferably you need a partner who respects your need for freedom, variety and self-expression. Within this framework, the following essences can assist you positively in helping you promise real allegiance and pledge loyalty.

Dedication....

Many-Headed Dryandra essence focuses on bringing fulfilment together with the consistent commitment needed in a longterm relationship. It instils interest in developing relationships and the dedication and responsibility to maintain them.

Settling down....

Characteristically the traveller and the wanderer, you can find it hard enough to settle down physically, yet alone commit to a relationship. **Sweet Pea** essence helps you find your place on Earth and form bonds and connections with others.

Commitment....

The aptly-named **Wedding Bush** is helpful if you have trouble committing to a relationship or if your inconsistency actually sabotages the satisfaction you seek with others. This essence is helpful either in binding attachments within an existing affiliation or in helping an individual resist going from one relationship to another. It is also useful in bringing dedication to a goal or life-purpose.

Forming bonds....

If inadequate mothering or abandonment are issues in your life, this often manifests as an avoidance of emotional contact or an inability to commit. **Evening Primrose** essence helps heal early painful memories, assisting you to open up emotionally and to form deep emotional bonds with another.

Fidelity....

Deepening your connections with others, **Pearly Everlasting** is the essence to inspire devotion and fidelity. Sabina Pettit writes, 'this remedy can be especially helpful to those who feel unwilling and/or unable to make a deep and lasting commitment in relationship'. Her affirmation for this essence is 'I am committed to this process of growing together in love and harmony'.

> *'I am not afraid to pledge my devotion and to promise my commitment and loyalty'*

Careless with words

As a straight-talking Sagittarian, you can be relied upon to say exactly what is on your mind. Without intending to do so, though, you may offend others when you speak the truth bluntly or put something across in a tactless manner. Thinking before you speak helps improve relationship discord and enables you to interact with increased diplomacy, kindness and consideration for others.

Sensitivity.... **Kangaroo Paw** essence is for the Sagittarian who is insensitive or unaware of how their words or actions might affect others. Helping you to say the right thing at the right time, this essence makes it possible for you to relate with sensitivity.

Intention.... Relationships can be strengthened and communications improved with **Bush Gardenia** essence. In addition to helping instil a healthy, loving relationship with oneself and others, this essence also brings awareness of how to convey words so that they will be perceived in the manner in which they are intended.

Diplomacy.... The Sagittarian enthusiasm to share their knowledge with others can often result in them becoming self-righteous and autocratic. The essence of **Willowherb** balances your will with the force of your personality, ensuring that an individual is empowered and yet conducts interactions with others with humility and diplomacy.

Integrity.... The essence **Blue Delphinium** assists you to communicate effectively, with truth and integrity. It helps you to listen, both to others and to how you feel within yourself, so that you can respond in a straightforward manner, but peacefully and thoughtfully.

> *'I speak the words of my highest intention'*

My way is best!

The Sagittarian who believes that their truth is the only truth can be fanatical, narrow-minded and dogmatic. Aroused and with burning feelings of justice, you can be over-zealous and domineering at times. Eager to share and teach your knowledge, you are a motivating and inspiring speaker, but on occasions you can benefit from the value of silence and using wisdom with your words.

Contentment.... *Hibbertia* essence is not only helpful if you are the type that is addicted to gaining knowledge, it is also for individuals who thinks they know it all or who need always to be right. Creating a more desirable balance between the mind and the heart, this essence helps integrate intuition with ideas and rationality. It improves flexibility in thinking, increases contentment with your own knowledge and reduces judgmental attitudes and feelings of superiority.

Tolerance.... Breaking through rigid thinking and narrow-mindedness, **Freshwater Mangrove** essence helps you open up to new concepts, ideas and beliefs. This essence shifts prejudice or bigotry, replacing them with acceptance, tolerance and the ability to accept differences.

Understanding.... The eager Sagittarian can enthuse others with their ideals, but doing so may be interpreted as domination. The 'know-it-all' Sagittarian does not find it easy to listen to the thoughts and ideas of others. Believing that it is only their beliefs that are true can make them dogmatic or self-righteous. This condescending attitude may inhibit the formation of harmonious relationships. **Yellow Leschenaultia** essence increases one's sensitivity to accommodate the opinions of others and the humility to realize that you can learn by listening to others, whoever they may be.

Open-minded.... **Vervain** essence encourages the Sagittarian who assumes that his ideas are best or her beliefs the only right ones in the direction of permitting others to have their own opinions, without feeling threatened themselves. Helping you to see things from a wider perspective, this essence encourages openmindedness, so you no longer need to impose strong opinions on others. Encouraging a balanced manner, it enhances your natural warmth and spontaneity, enabling you to give much positive encouragement and inspiration to others.

> *'I respect the opinions and ideas of others'*

Kindhearted Sagittarius is generous and giving, but some types like to do things in a big way. Their 'over the top' style can involve recklessness. If you are never satisfied or restless, you may always be thinking that there is something or someone better. Being master of your passions and sensual natures restricts any excessive pleasure-loving behaviour that results in indulgence.

Restraint....

A tendency to sexual excess or overindulgence in food can be alleviated with the help of **Almond** essence. Lila Devi calls **Almond** 'The Self-container', because it promotes the qualities of moderation and self-discipline. Its balancing energy instils a wholesome sexuality and behaviour that is sexually well-adjusted. Lila Devi says, 'No, **Almond** essence does not weaken, repress or annihilate sexual energy; rather, it allows us to transmute this powerful force'. **Almond** helps with temperance on all levels not just sexual.

In perspective....

Inflating the facts or overstating and embroidering the truth? If you have a tendency to exaggerate, embellish or create a sense of drama in order to draw attention to yourself, **Woolly Smokebush** essence reduces this preoccupation with the self and allows you to see yourself with objectivity and without glamour. It helps provide the right perspective on yourself.

Humility....

Arrogant behaviour or a tendency to overestimate can be tempered with **Gymea Lily** essence. This essence instils humility and creates an awareness and appreciation of others and their contributions in any circumstance.

Moderation....

In addition to moderating extravagance, wastefulness and recklessness, **Philotheca** essence also works to balance any situation where an individual feels blocked from receiving love, appreciation or acknowledgment from others.

Control....

Whether it is over-eating, addictions or obsessive behaviour, then **Blue China Orchid** essence strengthens the will to break old habits, helping any astrological sign—not just Sagittarius—to create new healthier patterns.

> *'My experiences are always balanced and
> I do everything in moderation'*

Resolving possible physical imbalances

☛ See p. 12
on how the
essences work

Please note that throughout this book suggestions of a medical nature are not in any way claiming that the essences will cure disease, and should not be followed as a substitute to consulting a qualified medical practitioner.

The liver

The liver is crucial in detoxifying impurities in the bloodstream and in absorbing nutrients from the blood. According to Debbie Shapiro, 'The liver is known as the seat of anger, a place where anger is stored, for keeping the blood clean can mean having to extract the negativity from it. Liver disorders often give rise to depression, which can be seen as anger turned towards ourselves'. The importance of *Blue Lupin* essence is in its ability to purify emotions such as anger, frustration and depression. It cleanses and detoxifies both on a mental and physical level. In addition to resolving feelings of irritability and anger, the sea essence *Mussel* promotes the flow of bile, which is secreted by the liver.

The benefit of *Dagger Hakea* essence is that it facilitates forgiveness, so you do not hold on to any anger and bitterness—thus assisting the health of the liver. Useful for removing negativity and unhelpful repetitive thoughts, *Plantain* essence is also useful for blood and liver disorders.

The lower back and pelvis

Dr Christine Page links the hips to stability in movement. She writes that 'disharmony relates to the inability to move forward confidently whether due to fear or feelings of insecurity'. *Dog Rose* essence addresses fears and insecurities, instilling courage to enable an individual to move ahead with confidence. Ian White (ABFH) suggests this essence, together with *Crowea* and *Spinifex*, for sciatica. *Crowea* has a beneficial action on the muscles in the body, which in this case may be tightened and contributing to nerve discomfort. He also writes that '*Spinifex* can be considered if there has been damage to nerve endings anywhere in the body'.

Two essences from the Pacific range address this lower back and pelvic area. Treating blocked energy or injury to the sacrum or pelvic girdle, *Candystick* essence can be considered. Workings on the bones, muscles, fascia and spinal alignment, *Salmonberry* essence enhances structural balancing.

Addictions and dependencies

In addition to establishing pattern and routine in one's life, *Morning Glory* essence is also helpful for any addictive habits. It reduces nervousness and restlessness. Restoring self-awareness and a healthy sense of ego, *Milkweed* essence imparts the strength and self-reliance to cope with any dependencies, so you are able to manage the demands and responsibilities of normal life. *Forsythia* essence works on any unhelpful patterns of behaviour, habits or addictions that are holding you back. It provides the motivation, strength and willingness to break and conquer alcohol, drug, tobacco or similar addictions.

10. THE CAPRICORN OUTLOOK ON LIFE AND HEALTH

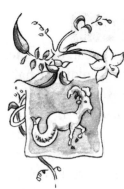

Capricorn

December 22–
January 21

Quality & element:
Cardinal Earth

Ruler: Saturn

Opposite sign:
Cancer

Soul-lesson: Love

CONSTITUTION

CAPRICORN'S hardworking outlook on life is nothing if not admirable. It is important for Capricornians to build, plan, structure or achieve on some level, and they tend to do this with unwavering strength and great tenacity. Their determination and dedication to hard work makes them extremely enduring; they stop for nothing and are undeterred by anybody. As Capricorn is a cardinal sign, they instigate and activate rather than accept things, and as an earth sign they are totally realistic and practical in their actions. In addition to being very dependable, they bear responsibility well and make good, fair managers, organizers or administrators. They can provide others with sound advice, and make loyal, sincere and reliable friends, although they can be hard on themselves and others at times in their attempt to attain their goals.

Usually conservative in their outlook, Capricornians are private and place a high value on security and home. In spite of being deeply committed to loved ones, they are not usually emotional but like nothing more than to be admired and respected.

Implications for health

The Capricornian often finds it difficult to express feelings or to react with much of an outward display of affection, something which may adversely affect his or her moods. Suppressed emotions may also build up in the skeletal framework of the Capricorn's body, perhaps manifesting as aches and pains, stiff joints, arthritis or rheumatism, and sometimes affecting physical mobility. It is beneficial for these people to try and maintain flexibility in their thinking, otherwise a closed or unyielding way of thinking can result in physical rigidity. The importance of the letting go of extreme self-will, pride or inflexible thinking, which can manifest as arthritis, is emphasized by Debbie Shapiro. She writes the following about arthritis. 'There can be a sense of being tied down, restricted, restrained and confined; also a developing inability to bend, to be mentally flexible or to be able to surrender. This can reflect a lack of self-trust as well as a hardening attitude toward life'.

The skin can be a problem area for Capricornians, and as the skin reflects how one feels about oneself, it can be seen as a boundary between one and the outside world. Capricornians' reputations are important to them, for they are concerned about how other people view them. If they react adversely to trauma and stress or have an inability to cope with the behaviour of others, these feelings can literally get under their skin. So too can Capricornians suffer with hearing problems, when they create boundaries and do not listen to others or to their inner selves. It is advisable that Capricorns take care of their teeth also.

Situated beneath the liver is the gall bladder, a possibly vulnerable area for a Capricorn. It is the reservoir for bile (produced by the liver) and its job is to emulsify fats so that they can be digested and absorbed by the body. Bile is representative of angry feelings such as frustration, bitterness and resentment. In their eagerness to achieve and let nothing stand in their way, some Capricorns adopt hardened and negative attitudes to life. These types of thought-patterns, according to Debbie Shapiro, 'can congeal and harden, becoming gallstones, that may be very painful to release'. There are further notes on these conditions at the end of the chapter.

HEALING AND SELF-DEVELOPMENT
FOR CAPRICORNIANS

The mind

If you are a Capricorn, then your intent and resolve are outstanding qualities, but at times they can make you inflexible and uncompromising. This rigidity may materialize in your vulnerable areas, as stiffness in the knees and other joints. Louise Hay believes that the knee is connected to one's pride and ego. The proud Capricorn can find it difficult to yield or bend in certain situations, and this often means they have lessons to learn in becoming more accepting and surrendering to a higher authority than themselves. If you are such a one, you may find that this higher authority is an external power or some inner aspect of yourself you tend to deny or not recognize.

Pragmatic and realistic in your thinking, you would be well advised to pay attention to your feelings and learn to use your intuition more. Remaining adaptable and open to new ideas is extremely beneficial to the Capricornian, who can find that being close-minded and uncompromising crystalllizes the mind and body. An accommodating attitude will increase your ability to move forward in life, and as your journey becomes smoother, your knees bend and your body becomes more flexible.

The body

Outdoor activities can be very therapeutic and enjoyable for Capricorn people, and they often enjoy rugged sports such as hillwalking and mountain-climbing.

As Capricorn rules the bony framework of the body, it is important for you to maintain the structure, correct condition and stance for your body. Alexander Technique is an excellent choice to follow in maintaining or correcting postures. Yoga, with its attention to the breath, can be a helpful way of releasing tension at the same time as keeping the body stretched and supple. Treatments such as osteopathy and chiropractic are often of benefit to Capricorn people if problems do occur. A natural form of healing energy can be sought through the use of crystals and gems, with which Capricorn has an affinity. This can derive through the actual wearing of crystals on the body, understanding how to place them appropriately within your home, or by treatment from an actual therapist. You also need to be reminded to take time for yourself, to rest and enjoy a bit of pampering at times.

☞ Read the Cancer chapter too—your opposite sign.

The spirit

USING YOUR INNER POWER AND FINDING YOUR SPIRITUAL MISSION

The influence of Saturn, Capricorn's ruling planet, is associated with authority and responsibility and may be the reason so many Capricorn people are found in positions of influence and command. It can however mean that you are strict and demanding of yourself and may even deny yourself the simple pleasures in life. Your great strength of purpose, together with your determination and discipline, positions you well for service in the world, which is your soul-lesson. Before you can influence others or respond to the call of authority, you need to learn to listen to your own inner voice and establish your inner authority and self-respect. Time spent on inner development and reflection will ensure that your inner power and strength manifest positively rather than just for self-preservation or gain. As you learn maturity and wisdom, you are able to realize the impermanence of worldly achievements, which may have impressed the young Capricorn. Your sense of authority, together with your acceptance of responsibility and duty, is superbly employed in serving others or in some service to your community.

☞ For the Soul-lessons, see pp. 13 & 25

SUGGESTED ESSENCES FOR CAPRICORNIANS

Resolving possible personality imbalances

As a Capricorn, you are patient, enduring and prepared to work hard for whatever you want. Your huge willpower and persistent spirit enables you to handle obstacles and set-backs. However, unfounded fears can hold you back and rigid views or pessimistic attitudes can inhibit your growth and progress. Your reserved and restrained nature does not always allow you to be in touch with your emotional side.

Acknowledging and releasing suppressed feelings

Cool, calm and collected, a typical Capricorn is unlikely to react with any great passion! In fact you can find it hard to express your innermost emotions and often deny your feelings. Any flamboyant and extreme displays of emotion from others are likely to distance you further from your own.

Cut off from emotions....

The essence **Bluebell** (AB) awakens suppressed feelings and can assist when you feel totally cut off from your emotions. It works on keeping the heart open and creating a consciousness of abundance, which encourages you to let go of fear and be more loving and giving.

Denying feelings....

Ideal for the typical Capricorn who is led by their head, not their heart, the rose essence **Marie Pavie** provides the confidence for you to follow your heart and not deny what you feel inside. It is also encouraging if you have suffered deep disappointment in relationships.

Sharing feelings....

The positive qualities of **Flannel Flower** essence enable you to express open, sensitive and gentle feelings in your physical and emotional interactions with others. Enhancing the ability to share, it is valuable if you do not feel comfortable with your feelings, if you experience difficulty in communicating emotions, or if you tend to draw away from physical closeness.

True feelings.... Helping you to recognize your true feelings, **Honesty** essence provides you with the ability to express yourself freely. Often, being critical of yourself can leave you fearing judgment and criticism from others. This essence reduces this sensitivity, loosens up reserved natures and liberates repressed emotions.

Breaking barriers.... The essence **Grass of Parnassus** is ideal if you tend to form protective barriers to shield yourself from emotional vulnerability or fear. It helps you more easily to release cut-off emotions and to share your feelings more easily with others.

> '*I am comfortable with my emotions, and it is safe for me to express my feelings*'

Overcoming fears

If you are anxious about not having enough in life, you may see life very gravely. The reserved or over-cautious Capricorn can place personal security and status high on their list, whereas there are others who are so fearful, usually of material or worldly events, that this can paralyze them with insecurities.

Fear.... **Mimulus** essence can release you from such fears; it brings balance, inner strength and the courage to face the world. It can restore your sense of determination, enabling you to withstand all manner of limitations and restriction in pursuit of your goals.

Terror.... Supplying feelings of peace and a soothing sense of not being alone in the world, **Red Clover** essence provides support if you are a fearful Capricornian. Sensitive to the events and happenings going on around you, it is easy for you to become terrified and alarmed. Comforting and reassuring, this essence sustains and nourishes you with a protective feeling of calm.

Nameless dread.... The saying for **Ribbon Pea** essence is 'Safe within the universe' (Barnao). Feelings of apprehension, anxiety and foreboding are quelled by this essence, as it helps liberate you from deep dread, terror or panic. Its positive energy is calming and composing, so you can conquer any fears of the unknown and go forward in life with serenity.

Overawed.... Empowering an individual with inner strength, **Thistle** essence provides resilience if you feel overawed by difficulties or challenges. Instilling confidence where fear existed before, it enables you to react in a self-assured manner and take firm action.

> *'I am safe, secure and always protected'*

You can do it!

Although not all Capricornians are high achievers, it is in their nature to be keen for success or accomplishment on some level. However, when overwhelmed or discouraged by challenges and hardships, you can become disillusioned. Feelings of failure can creep in and hold you back from accomplishing your goals, not to mention diminishing your energy. You can benefit from encouragement and praise from others in order to motivate yourself.

Inner strength.... Providing you with the inner strength to succeed and a success consciousness, **Woolly Banksia** essence increases your enthusiasm and supplies the determination needed for you to reach your goals. It replaces heavy, resigned and disparaged states with hope, strength and the vitality to face any adversities in life.

Incentive.... Living up to its name, **Passionate Life** essence is a combination created from *Amaryllis Belladonna*, Apophyllite, pale amerthyst and and clear quartz. It supplies stimulus and incentive, especially when you are living your life narrowly. This motivating essence not only increases energy and zest for life but also provides the courage and confidence to cope with obstructions, setbacks or obstacles.

Acceptance.... If you are at a point of despair, when things look so grim that it seems that they are never going to go right, then **Sweet Hunza** essence brings acceptance of the situation. Helping you to see the reason behind an experience and the opportunity associated with it, this essence triggers the realization that however hard the experience, it is meant to be. Ultimately, good will prevail.

> *'I have the strength to endure and the motivation to succeed'*

Feeling stuck and frustrated?

Typically conventional and conformist, you tend to stick with established order. This enables you to be realistic and practical but it can inhibit your ability to embrace anything unusual or new. If you feel stuck or frustrated, this is a signal for you to open up a bit and take a fresh approach to things.

Flexibility....

In addition to removing rigidity and resistance to change, **Bauhinia** essence increases flexibility and tolerance. Inspiring you to consider new approaches, views and concepts, it encourages you to become less narrow and more accepting of different people and situations.

Inherited patterns....

Maybe as a result of family conditioning, Capricorn's nature can be to inhibit you or hold you back. **Boab** is a powerful essence, strong enough to break through any inherited habits or belief-patterns that are not serving your best interests. With its assistance, you are able to release any unhelpful or negative thoughts and take your own course of action without feeling trapped by generational standards or family precedent. Rather than obeying longstanding or established expectations, you are free to do what is right for *you*!

Purpose....

Capricorn likes to have a purpose, and when you do not know what to do with yourself you can become directionless and feel worthless. In addition to establishing purpose, persistence and perseverance, **Kapok Bush** essence provides a 'kick up the backside' for individuals who become disheartened and apathetic. Rather than accepting situations with resignation, this essence prompts you to take charge of your life once again.

Courage....

The saying for **Menzies Banksia** essence is 'To Live Again' (Barnao), and its energy is freeing and regenerating if you feel stuck or blocked. It helps you move through difficult situations or experiences and once again see the light. If you become immovable, caught up in past happenings, completely thwarted, frustrated and unable to act, then this essence rejuvenates, bringing optimism and joy. It instils the courage to move ahead fearlessly if you fear the repetition of uncomfortable past events.

> *'With an open mind, I move forward to embrace new opportunities and possibilities with ease'*

A little inner reflection

Many Capricornians focus on the material world and achieving, in order to secure wealth or reach the peak of their profession, yet do not always find the satisfaction they are seeking. As you mature, you may realize the shallowness of merely existing in the physical world, and that real wealth and power are to be found beyond the ego and the material world. By learning to look within, and by identifying with a higher consciousness or embracing a spiritual understanding of life, you are more likely to find fulfilment. In order to do so you need to be able to allow your perspective to rise out of purely earthly life and to feel safe with your intuition and feelings.

Trusting feelings....

An essence that helps you to become more in touch with your intuition and to trust your gut feelings is **Bush Fuchsia**. It also increases your confidence to be able to speak out about your own convictions.

Deeper perceptions....

Assisting individuals with a purely material perspective to move away from this stance is the essence **Bush Iris**. Enhancing spiritual awareness, this essence is also useful in a meditative practice, to deepen perceptions and visualizations.

Awareness....

Your ruling planet, Saturn, is the tester and the teacher, and it can push Capricorn people to the limit of their endurance. **Mint Bush** essence not only provides you with the ability to cope on these occasions, but it also enables an awareness of spirituality to emerge during stressful times. This essence helps you to view restrictions and limitations in your life as opportunities to make progress on a deeper inner level. **Mint Bush** also supports those of you who feel at times that their values are shifting and the structures of life seems to be crumbling and falling away.

> *'My inward perspective enables me to understand my lessons in my life and to find inner fulfilment'*

Balancing Capricorn energy

Saturn teaches patience, responsibility, duty and determination. Its influence often means that it is through tests, delays, difficulties and limitation that you learn wisdom and humility. This means that you often see life as an uphill battle and the importance of rising above earthly limitations and keeping a positive attitude is essential for you. Owing to your very earthbound perspective, you can easily fall into darkness and pessimism, which can sometimes manifest as ill-health or limiting circumstances. You can benefit from focusing on positive thoughts and keeping in mind the saying that 'energy follows thought'.

Weighed down with life

When responsibilities weigh heavily and your tendency is to succumb to gloom, melancholy and depression, the following essences are uplifting.

Joy....

Red Rose essence is for negative thoughts and for the many causes of depression. Sabina Pettitt writes about finding the joy within, with this essence: 'Joy will no longer depend on external conditions but will come from the internal spring of Joy which dwells in each of us'. Her jubilant affirmation for this essence is 'I am the Joy of a full bloom' (THF).

Vitality....

The essence **Cucumber** can be used to rebalance an individual during times of depression. If you feel detached from life, then this essence replaces any sadness and dejection with increased vitality and a desire to reintegrate into life.

Upliftment....

Releasing from negativity, the essence of **Orange** uplifts despairing, apathetic and resigned states. This essence is energizing and it renews enthusiasm and interest in life so that you have the power to endure setbacks and obstacles on your climb to the top of the mountain. Lila Devi writes, '**Orange** trumpets hope and leads us through even the most longterm suffering to the light at the end of the tunnel'.

Self-recognition....

You like to feel recognized for your efforts, and when this appreciation is not forthcoming from others you can become despondent and 'down'. **Yellow Cone Flower** essence helps you to recognize yourself as valued and esteemed, thus ensuring that you do not rely on approval or appreciation from others. This essence instils values of self-importance and positive worth, regardless of outside validation.

> 'My life is a joy'

Looking on the bright side

Exceedingly realistic, practical and quite introspective, you may sometimes benefit from a little lightening up, particularly if you become downbeat in your thinking. The pessimistic Capricorn, especially, can have a perception of life that is full of fearful anticipation. Often straining to fulfil obligations, with your strong sense of duty (especially towards work) you do not always allow for much pleasure, fun or frivolity in your life.

All is well....

Red Clover essence encourages you to have a positive view of life without worry and anxiety. Its comforting energy reassures the sensitive Capricorn and provides a secure base from which you can approach life.

Cheerful....

If your tendency is to sombreness, this can make life more challenging and difficult for you. Your ability to see from a perspective of fun and goodwill, even in difficult and stressful situations, can be restored by **Yellow Flag Flower** essence. It helps you to remain strong, cheerful and untroubled, despite everyday pressures or worries.

Simplicity....

The words that sum up **Spinach** essence are 'simplicity', 'uncomplicated' and 'freeing'. This essence replaces fear, worry and overwhelmed states with carefree humour. It helps you to see life simply, without complication and from a more childlike and playful perspective. For the Capricorn who is overconscious of status and prestige, this essence also eliminates these illusionary and pretentious states, encouraging an appreciation of nature and the fundamental things in life.

Optimism.... The cheerful and optimistic energy of **Wild Violet** essence enhances your enjoyment of life. If your overcautious nature means that you miss out on opportunities because of anxiety and fear, this essence imbues a positive attitude, permitting you to embrace the future without worry.

> *'I choose to see my life with lightness and optimism'*

Inner strength

The following essences awaken in you the necessary strength to keep climbing your mountains.

Staying power.... **Waratah** essence provides the staying power to endure any manner of difficult circumstances you may encounter in your life. It enhances courage and the resolve to cope at trying times. In addition to supplying determination and fortitude, **Waratah** is very powerful in times of depression and hopelessness.

Empowering.... Instilling belief in oneself, the empowering essence **Tomato** enables you to overcome challenges and setbacks that may arise. Replacing a defeatist attitude with one of success and hope, this essence imparts willpower, together with an unshakeable and unbeatable faith in oneself. Not only providing the conviction for you to fight your battles, it also resolves any fear or terror that can impede you from achieving your goals.

Strengthening.... If there are times when the dedicated and dependable Capricorn becomes overwhelmed and exhausted by overwork or responsibility, then **Elm** essence encourages and strengthens your purpose. Resolving feelings of inadequacy and doubt in your abilities, this essence provides awareness of your own capabilities and enables you to see things in proportion.

Realism.... Individuals requiring **Oak** essence are patient and committed, but will struggle on against all difficulties and at any cost, often to their own detriment. If you are the type that never gives in or has an unrealistic expectation of your performance, endurance and invincibility, this essence helps break down this fixed, unforgiving attitude. It throws attention onto over-commitment to duty by encouraging flexibility, together with a realistic output of your efforts, and increased enjoyment of life.

Relax and lighten up

*Have fun with the following essences, especially if you deny
spontaneity or tend to be sober or too solemn!*

Fun....

For these times, **Valerian** essence can lift your spirits, instil a
sense of fun and give you back your sense of humour. It is
inspiring if you are overly responsible and weighed down by
cares, worries or overwork.

Play....

Little Flannel Flower is the essence of fun and playfulness, and
its ability to establish a carefree and untroubled mood is useful
when you take yourself too seriously.

Humour....

Blackberry's uplifting qualities elevate your thoughts and increase your sense of humour. This essence also bestows a purity of thought at times when your mind is closed, judgmental,
negative or critical. It enables you to think optimistically, hope-
fully and cheerfully.

Enjoyment....

Confirming self-acceptance and self-esteem, **Vanilla Leaf** essence encourages you to find joy and self-belief. It inspires you
to rejoice in being unique and special.

Laughter....

In FLOWERS THAT HEAL, Judy Griffin's affirmation for **Wild Oats**
(PF) essence is 'Laughter is my medicine'. She writes about this
essence, 'We can easily let go and laugh our way past imperfec-
tions and inhibitions holding back natural growth'.

Expectations of oneself

*Always trying to live up to the high standards you set for
yourself, the typical Capricorn is not usually content with
him- or herself or his–her efforts. Continual striving and over-*

conscientiousness can produce tiredness and depression.

Self-acceptance....

In addition to enhancing your sense of joy in life, **Pine** essence instils a healthy self-recognition and self-satisfaction, together with pragmatic expectations and goals.

Open-minded....

The 'loosening up' essence **Rock Water** frees you from excessive self-discipline, perfectionism or the tendency to deny your own needs. Encouraging an openminded and a flexible attitude, this essence enables you to enjoy yourself more and take pleasure in life.

Self-liberating....

Fig essence transforms overly serious, overly disciplined or inhibited natures. Its relaxing qualities instil self-worth and self-liberation, so you do not place unrealistic expectations upon yourself. Inspiring a flexible 'go with the flow' attitude, this essence helps you become less rigid, self-critical or self-denying.

Self-worth....

Judy Griffin (FTH) recommends the essence **Basil** in the following terms. 'This personality would consider himself and his achievements not good enough. Oftentimes, this person is a perfectionist with an inferiority complex'. *Basil* essence increases self-worth, and is especially useful to you if you measure your merit by financial success alone.

> *'I am happy with myself and my best is always good enough'*

Relating and communicating

Our relationships with others can either enhance our lives or make them very difficult. How we get on with others can be a measure of how we feel about and get on with ourselves. The challenges of life can result in hardened and cynical attitudes, which can adversely affect your relationships with people. If you are reluctant to get involved with the problems of others, this can make you seem impersonal and detached. In your attempt to be well thought-of and respected, others may sometimes perceive you as cold or calculating. This rough exterior can make it appear that you do not get hurt, yet underneath you can be vulnerable and find it difficult to ask others for help. If you are an inflexible Capricorn, believing that your way is best, and like always to be right, then your great pride does not make it easy for you to admit defeat or acknowledge that you can be in the wrong sometimes.

Keeping the heart open

Tenderness....   If life has been tough and you feel wounded or hurt, the essence *Orange Leschenaultia* prevents you from closing up emotionally or creating barriers round yourself. This essence establishes softness and tenderness, so you are able to relate with sincerity and compassion towards yourself and others.

Sadness....   Having the power to release past pains and sadness from your psyche, the essence *Sturt Desert Pea* enables you to let go of grief and sorrow. It discharges bottled-up or painful feelings, enabling you to communicate more freely.

Compassion....   The toughening up that can result from some life-experiences may make some Capricornians austere, unfeeling and unsympathetic in order to protect themselves. *Rough Bluebell* essence addresses this indifference or the conscious intent you may have to cut off love from others. It helps when you have distanced yourself from feelings and emotions and have forgotten how to express love. This essence heals by instilling kindness, compassion and sensitivity where the needs of others are important.

Receptivity....   If you find it difficult to express affection or to open up to closeness in relationships, the essence of *Red Leschenaultia* heightens sensitivity, receptivity and intimacy. Any cynical, disapproving or unsentimental feelings towards others are de-energized by this essence, as it replaces cold and unsympathetic feelings with gentleness, trust and kindness.

Cautiousness....   Judy Griffin's affirmation (FTH) for the rose essence *Cecil Brunner* is 'I feel safe to bloom'. It helps the cautious Capricorn to feel comfortable enough to enter into a new relationship without restraint. Also assisting in overcoming fears, this essence makes it easier to tackle challenges and any new situations.

> *'I am gentle and sensitive with myself and others'*

Interacting and sharing with others

Your quiet demeanour and self-sufficient manner can make it appear to others that you are a loner—which can be true to a certain extent. You do need others but you are reserved and cautious about commitment (but extremely loyal having done so) and very concerned about getting hurt, which can isolate you further.

Increasing closeness....

Enabling you to share your feelings with others and express your emotions with warmth, **Flannel Flower** essence assists if you feel vulnerable, uneasy or fearful of mixing with others. This essence embodies gentleness and sensitivity, making it possible for you to be comfortable with closeness or physical touching.

Detrimental feelings....

Boab essence not only helps you release yourself from any detrimental family traits and habits, it also enables you to let go of any deeply-held emotions that you may find hard to express or that you have been indoctrinated to keep inside.

Social skills....

If you hold back or feel cut off from others, **Yellow Cowslip Orchid** essence can increase your social skills and encourage you to integrate and interact with greater ease. In addition to reducing overly-intellectual approaches or the tendency to judge or criticize, it lessens the typical Capricornian tendency to adhere to rigid petty routines or bureaucracy.

Belonging....

According to Ian White (ABFE), **Tall Yellow Top** essence is 'the remedy for isolation and loneliness'. He writes that 'it is also for the lack of love as Tall Yellow Top helps to re-connect the head and the heart'. Instilling a sense of belonging, it helps if you experience low self-esteem or feelings of separation from others, especially if you are without a job or some sort of work to identify with.

Being comfortable....

If you feel uncomfortable mixing with other people or tend to be the loner, the essence **Tall Mulla Mulla** helps to overcome this discomfort. Rather than allowing you to feel withdrawn or ill at ease, it helps you to enjoy social interactions and to feel secure with others.

> *'I feel confident and comfortable in the company of other people'*

The overly serious Capricorn can come across sternly in front of others. Defensive and sometimes narrow in their views, they can at times be a law unto themselves!

Consider-
ation....

Increasing tolerance and sensitivity, **Beech** essence transforms any limited, restrictive belief-patterns or judgments you may hold of others. Opening you up to a higher aspect of yourself, this essence reduces inner rigidity and encourages easiness, sympathy and consideration for others and their views.

Understand-
ing....

Yellow Leschenaultia essence can also improve relationships by encouraging renewed openness, broad-mindedness and consideration for the opinions of others. If you are looking to be more concerned, sensitive or tolerant of others, this essence enhances understanding, acceptance and increased interest in other people.

Forgiveness....

In addition to facilitating an open expression of your feelings, **Dagger Hakea** essence transforms any feelings of resentment or bitterness, even if these feelings are buried and you are not necessarily aware of the importance of forgiveness in order to move on in life.

Compassion....

Intolerant and unaccepting natures are transformed with **Date** essence, as it inspires qualities of compassion and sensitivity. It helps increase your warmth and acceptance of others, so that you become more receptive and open, which encourages others to be naturally drawn towards you.

> *'I let go of perfection and judgment and see others with understanding'*

Inner authority

Although you can have high expectations of others, you are mostly fair and just. If these traits get out of balance, though, you can be a hard taskmaster; your behaviour can be demanding—even dictatorial and authoritarian.

Wise power....   ***Rose Alba*** essence brings about a balanced and wise expression of your power and leadership abilities. It also moderates the behaviour of those individuals who can be strictly conventional, overly traditional or proud—who may withhold emotions or withdraw from expressing themselves.

Modesty....   ***Gymea Lily*** essence instils a balanced use of one's power, tempering dominating and controlling behaviour with a more modest approach and a consideration for others. It establishes humility if a desire to be recognized for your efforts results in attention or status-seeking. Its powerful, strong energy empowers you to achieve and fulfil your goals, at the same time helping you to resolve any issues around authority or authority figures.

Respect....   In addition to helping increase self-respect, ***Yellow Hyacinth*** essence generates a healthy respect for others and an appreciation of their unique qualities. It also conquers any feelings of superiority or arrogance arising out of a lack of self-esteem.

Confidence....   Named 'The Confident One', ***Pineapple*** essence infuses your being with a strong sense of identity and personal power, yet a sense that is blended with good judgment. In her book, Lila Devi connects ***Pineapple*** essence with abundance and money issues—a subject quite close to most Capricornians' hearts. She writes the following about the negative ***Pineapple*** state (i.e., someone needing this essence), 'a self-fulfilling prophecy of defeat in which we might feel underpaid or unrecognized for our achievements.' 'These circumstances are often mere reflections of our own poor self-image'. With the assistance of this essence, feelings of inferiority or dissatisfaction with oneself may make way for self-content, fulfilment and graciousness. It helps the shy Capricorn become more self-assured and the proud Capricorn acquire a modest wisdom.

> *'I am self-assured and I treat others*
> *with respect and consideration'*

Resolving possible physical imbalances

☞ *See p. 12 on how the essences work*

Note that suggestions of a medical nature are not in any way claiming a cure of disease, and should not be followed as a substitute to consulting a qualified medical practitioner.

Skin deep

Judy Griffin believes that personalities who do not feel good about themselves can manifest their beliefs in a physical condition, such as a skin problem. In FLOWERS THAT HEAL she advises *Salvia* essence to enhance a positive self-image and also to improve skin conditions.

In addition to enforcing a strong sense of self-approval, *Vanilla Leaf* essence also works physically on the skin. Aptly named for Capricorn, *Billy Goat Plum* essence is also beneficial for skin problems. If feelings of oneself are of revulsion or abhorrence, this essence heals this state and the skin afflictions that these feelings may materialize.

Physical stiffness

Little Flannel Flower is the essence of fun and playfulness, and its ability to establish a carefree and untroubled mood can be instrumental in alleviating physical stiffness.

The challenges that *Snowdrop* (PAC) essence addresses are 'Fear and Restriction' and the affirmation for it is 'I can let go and experience joy'. According to Sabina Pettitt, this essence 'strengthens the will and dissolves paralyzing fear'. 'It helps us get mobilized'. Embodying qualities of personal power, leadership and joyful enthusiasm, it is an essence that frees up energy blockages such as stiffness and arthritis, blockages that contribute to your freedom of physical expression.

Concentrating on the bones, muscles and fascia, the essence *Salmonberry* works on spinal alignment and structural balance. It helps release thoughts and feeelings that have contributed towards holding patterns in the body. *Pink Seaweed* essence addresses change and inflexibility by helping you adjust to changing conditions. Physically, it strengthens the bones and teeth and is also used for constipation. *Vine* essence supports the back by releasing inflexibility and tension in this area.

Ian White (ABFH) writes how effective *Gymea Lilly* essence is in working with problems in the bones and ligaments and how it is used by a number of osteopaths and chiropractors to align the spine. He also suggests the following flower essences for arthritis: *Bauhinia, Boab, Flannel Flower, Little Flannel Flower, Yellow Cowslip Orchid, Dagger Hakea* and *Sturt Desert Pea*. All these essences, mentioned earlier, work to clear destructive habits, sadness or bitterness and to facilitate a flexible, open, tolerant attitude and easy expression of one's feelings, and consequent physical improvement.

The gall bladder

Helping you let go of intense emotions, the essence *Pink Geranium* eases emotional pain and releases suppressed feelings, particularly of anger. It is healing for the liver and gallbladder, which can take the brunt of these feelings. Beneficial for both these organs and for dealing with feelings of irritation and frustration is the sea essence *Mussel.* It promotes the flow of bile and aids digestion. Judy Griffin (FTH) writes the following about *Garden Mum* essence. 'Critical and bitter thoughts may affect the liver and gall bladder, blocking energy otherwise used to secrete the enzyme bile, to separate fats.' She suggests this essence to help remove and lighten these blocks and to encourage the acceptance of everyone just as they are.

Ian White (ABFE) writes that *Dagger Hakea* essence 'primarily brings about the open expression of feelings and forgiveness'. It is particularly helpful if you are someone who keeps feelings of resentment and bitterness locked away inside, for to do so is thought to be instrumental in the creation of gallstones. He prescribes this essence to unblock the emotion that is causing the stones to form.

11. THE AQUARIUS OUTLOOK ON LIFE AND HEALTH

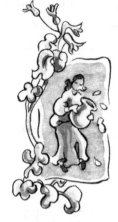

Aquarius

*January 21–
February 19*

*Quality & element:
Fixed air*

*Rulers: Saturn &
Uranus*

Opposite sign: Leo

*Soul-lesson:
Brotherhood*

CONSTITUTION

THE TYPICAL Aquarian is friendly, with an interest in everyone they encounter. Despite being gregarious and sociable, Aquarians have quite an impersonal and detached approach to life. It can be hard to pin them down; they greatly value their freedom and need to spend time alone, something that can bring a tendency to isolation. As they are so independent and tend not to rely on others or ask for their help, their solitude can sometimes result in their feeling lonely, depressed or remote from others.

Charmingly unique and individual, an Aquarian does things his or her way, which is often contrary to the norm. Be prepared for the unexpected with Aquarians! Yet their love for their fellow beings means that they are often motivated to use their talents to serve humanity. On a personal level, though, they may very much need love but often do not let others get close enough to give it. Like other subjects of air-element signs, they tend to live mainly in their heads. They are constantly thinking, analyzing and planning: enclosed in the activities of their minds. This level of mental focus can be draining, sometimes causing them to work themselves into a state of nervous exhaustion, while in the process they can cut themselves off from others.

Implications for health

Contrary to some people's assumptions, the wave symbol for Aquarius, which is known as 'the water bearer', does not make Aquarius a water sign. Rather, the symbol represents thought-waves and depicts the outpouring of collective consciousness. Aquarius is associated with universal knowledge; Aquarians' ideals and visions are often ahead of their time. These waves also portray electrical waves of pulsating energy and have much to do with the circulation of energy throughout the nervous system of the body.

It is somewhat of a contradiction that as a sign of fixed quality, Aquarius does not always embrace change easily and yet (because they may be among the most progressive and inventive thinkers) Aquarians are most often accepting of new concepts—implying an element of adaptability. This has much to do with the influence of the two planets that rule Aquarius. The planet Saturn is conventional and dutiful, as opposed to the forward-thinking and freedom-loving planet Uranus. A healthy Aquarian needs to incorporate a balance of both these principles in their lives.

These differing qualities can be linked physically to the Aquarius-ruled part of the body, the ankle. Dr Christine Page links the ankle with freedom of movement (related to Uranus) and she writes that disharmony here relates to a feeling of restriction (related to Saturn) in the direction that one wants to take. Troubles in this vulnerable area can express the blocked energy within this conflict. Aquarius also rules the lower leg and the circulation of the blood in the body, which is why its subjects can be disposed to varicose veins, phlebitis, arteriosclerosis, thrombosis, spasm and cramps.

For a sign so concerned with the social structure of humanity, it is perhaps surprising that Aquarius does not usually get overly involved emotionally. Aquarians' objective manner and detached way of caring is more appropriate to their humanitarian pursuits and endeavours than an over-sentimental approach, even though this does mean that they can easily become out of touch with their bodies and their own emotional needs. In their friendships, this manner enables them to give dispassionate support and help to their many close acquaintances, although it is helpful for Aquarians to have some particular trusted friends who can encourage them to release their emotions and speak about their own needs.

HEALING AND SELF-DEVELOPMENT FOR AQUARIANS

The mind

If you are an Aquarian, you probably enjoy the spirit of the group. Your *forte* in life arises out of involvement with others, whether in associations, organizations, and clubs, or maybe just in your wide circle of friends and acquaintances. Your humanitarian instincts often lead you to devote some of your time to the wellbeing of society, providing you with the opportunity to work toward the welfare of others. Your typically Aquarian rational and impersonal way of caring and your huge compassion for humanity are a potent combination.

Your incentive to serve a cause or an ideal and your loyalty to it can be second to none. This motivation often takes a scientific or artistic direction, and is more often than not altruistic in nature. You have the ability to use your inventive and ingenious mind to bring forth exciting new thoughts, concepts and ideas that may be instrumental in creating revolutionary change to the benefit of humankind. The more traditional Aquarian is able to structure and give form to these unique suggestions, but unconventional Aquarians are better working with others who can ground their ideas and make them workable. Developing some sort of control over your thoughts, rather than being in your head all the time, can be of great benefit to you, since being able to still the mind has a calming effect on the nervous system.

The body

Future-orientated and forward-thinking, you are usually open to anything new and different, so you are quite likely to turn to alternative treatments or complementary medi-

☛ Read the Leo chapter too— your opposite sign

cine in your search for health or to maintain wellbeing.

It is your mind rather than your body that occupies most of your energy, but physical movement is important to you and should be encouraged. Any form of exercise, such as walking, running or cycling, that benefits the lower leg, calves and ankles and keeps the circulation moving is essential. Since Aquarius is connected with the electrical flow of energy around the body, acupuncture is an excellent choice of treatment for you—and not only physically, for it also brings the body, mind and spirit into harmonious alignment.

Your concern for the welfare of others, together with your humanistic values and social ideals, mean that working mainly on a mental level you can easily lose sight of your emotional needs. Occasional treatments involving touch, such as a massage, will help you to integrate your mind and body, making you more aware of your feelings.

The spirit

USING YOUR INNER POWER AND FINDING YOUR SPIRITUAL MISSION

Aquarians can lose their power when they are fixed and dogmatic in their thinking. Often believing that only their views and opinions are correct, they can close themselves to other beliefs and ideas. In some cases, this tendency can be a result of how past conditioning has formed attitudes and ways of thinking. It is useful for everyone, not just Aquarians, to become aware of how childhood conditioning, past programming and indoctrination can limit and restrict us. As Aquarians grow in wisdom and maturity they can expand their thinking to appreciate other viewpoints.

☛ For the Soul-lessons, see pp. 13 & 25

Some Aquarians can be seen as distant because they can be completely unaware of another's needs on an individual basis. Brotherhood is Aquarius's soul-lesson (as it is with all the air signs) and Aquarians can best actuate this lesson by learning how to understand the needs of others.

In order to communicate with compassion, it helps to embrace the qualities of your opposite sign, Leo. Combining

Aquarius's humanistic values with Leo's wisdom of the heart makes an effective combination with which to distribute the message of brotherhood throughout humankind.

SUGGESTED ESSENCES FOR AQUARIANS

Resolving possible personality imbalances

As an Aquarian, you are friendly and sociable, with a strong independent streak and often a touch of delightful eccentricity, a certain uniqueness. However, your free spirit and self-sufficient manner can make it easy for others to perceive you as indifferent and remote. If these characteristics are taken to the extreme, Aquarian individuals can be rebellious, unpredictable, unreliable or non-committal, which tends further to separate and alienate them from others. More conservative Aquarians, however, may need support and encouragement to help them believe in and express their uniqueness and individuality.

Aloof and detached

You possess a proud, reserved and independent nature, but your self-reliance may create barriers between you and others, as you can be perceived as distant or sometimes aloof.

Feeling unloved....

Water Violet essence thaws out any remoteness or inaccessibility, helping you to approach others with ease and to be involved with and warmly received by them.

Feeling rejected....

The self-reliant qualities of **Illawarra Flame Tree** essence are for if you need to have other people around you, or feel rejected if you do not. Releasing this need to seek approval from others, this essence provides you with strength and confidence, together with the commitment and responsibility to develop your own potential.

Feeling uncomfortable socially....

If you feel uncomfortable mixing with other people or you tend to be the loner, the essence **Tall Mulla Mulla** helps you to overcome this discomfort. Rather than feeling withdrawn or ill at ease, this essence helps you to enjoy social interactions and to feel secure with others.

> *'I feel secure and accepted by others'*

Tempering the rebel

The typical Aquarian nature can range between very individual and quietly wilful to wildly rebellious! The rebellious type delights in nonconformity or reacting against tradition; the Aquarian often does things to shock. Needing the freedom to express yourself freely, you may enjoy dressing or acting outrageously in order to be noticed, especially when young.

Moderation....

If the tendency to rebel is excessive, detrimental to your relationships or alienating you further from others, then the essence of **Illawarra Flame Tree** tempers this behaviour. Not only when you experience feelings of rejection and alienation but more generally, this essence helps you with your sense of identity, so you do not rely on extreme states to attract attention.

Respect....

Red Helmet Orchid essence tempers a hot-headed or selfish attitude towards those in authority. It releases frustration and intolerance, replacing them with consideration and respect. This essence increases and enhances the Aquarian leadership qualities as well as bringing an expanded awareness and sensitivity for others.

Self-control....

The energy of **Almond** essence is one of moderation and balance. Calming radical or rebellious tendencies, this essence is for self-control and moderation. It heals anxiety, stress or frustration by helping you to use your time and energy more wisely.

Diplomacy....

The disruptive or unruly Aquarian may find it difficult to get along with others or find him- or herself becoming a loner. **Jasmine** essence promotes a different perspective on life, where diplomacy replaces opposition and conflict. This essence dissolves feelings of isolation and alienation, giving way to a peaceful and orderly acceptance of your environment.

> 'Secure in my uniqueness, I am sensitive
> and cooperative with others'

Stuck in thinking

Aquarians have keen minds and are usually free and broad in their thinking. Once these people form an opinion, though, they can become totally fixed.

Liberation....

Very appropriate if you are the more traditional Aquarian, stubbornly adhering to your principles and ideologies, the essence of **Pincushion Hakea** inspires your inquisitive mind to be free and open, at the same time as taking a discriminating and practical view of things. Vasudeva and Kadambii Barnao write the following about this essence. 'The middle way is to be prepared to keep our mind open to new developments and expansions in consciousness, and choose that which is the most lifegiving and positive, be it an old realization or a new one'· In addition to liberating rigid ideas in religious, political, scientific or esoteric beliefs, this essence also encourages you if you are fearful to venture forward.

Flexibility....

Together with removing rigidity and resistance to change, **Bauhinia** essence increases flexibility and tolerance. It encourages you to consider new approaches, views and concepts, enabling you to be less narrow in your beliefs and more accepting of different people and situations.

Healing divisions....

Freshwater Mangrove essence opens you up to perceive opportunities, experiences and ideas in a new way. It frees up the intolerant or 'pig-headed' Aquarian, prejudiced about what they believe in, particularly those things they have been taught and not personally experienced. Affording the opportunity to overcome unjustified beliefs, this essence also inspires the ability to resolve differences and to heal divisions and splits with others.

Expanding thinking....

The gem essence **Azurite** integrates thinking from a 'head only' perspective with physical expression. When the connection is

234 · CENTAURY FOR VIRGO, ROCK ROSE FOR PISCES

missing it may contribute to physical depletion and bone and joint problems, maybe to arthritis.

> *'I expand my thinking and my mind*
> *is open to anything new'*

Just be yourself

It is often the Aquarian principles, ideas or belief-systems that are contrary to or in opposition to the opinion of the masses. Yet more conformist Aquarians may have a fear of being judged and need encouragement to break away from convention or distance themselves from an arrangement that is not in their best interests.

Being fearless....

Sabina Pettit writes the following about **Grass Widow** essence. 'Emotionally it relates to the fear around letting go of the illusion of comfortable discomfort if we find ourselves in a belief system that does not have the support of mass consciousnesses.' Encouraging you to be yourself without fear of being judged, **Grass Widow** essence instils the principle of freedom, enabling you to examine your beliefs and release any limitations, even if you feel separate from the group or do not have the support of others.

Being unique....

The essence **Bluebell** (PAC) stimulates openness and communication if you feel different, fear being noticed or have trouble making yourself understood. Releasing fears and liberating old programmed patterns, this essence encourages expression of your inner being and uniqueness.

Being independent....

Accentuating individuality, **Aquilegia Columbine** essence enhances your ability to think and act independently of others. This essence helps if you need encouragement to convey your distinctive personality, rather than adopt the role that others have chosen for you.

Being original....

The image that springs to mind of the humble **Buttercup** flower is of it holding its head proudly up to receive the light, and this is exactly what the qualities of its essence instil. Bringing recognition especially for the individual who lacks self-esteem, this essence is ideal for the unconventional or 'alternative' individual who may not acknowledge their unusualness or originality. This essence helps you recognize and accept your own uniqueness by relieving the need to judge yourself against the conventional benchmarks of achievement and success.

Be myself....   *Gymea Lily* essence supplies support if you feel unusual or different from others. Promoting a strong sense of self, it helps you to be unaffected by other people's opinions or judgments. In addition to encouraging you to express your inimitable self, this essence instils humility, tempers arrogance and enhances your listening ability.

> *'I am comfortable with myself and*
> *I embrace my uniqueness'*

Go your own way

The following essences are helpful if you need encouragement to believe in yourself, do your own thing, or follow your own path.

I'll do it my way....   The saying for **Pink Impatiens** essence is 'The courage of the lone traveller' (Barnao). Assisting you to stand by the convictions of your heart regardless of whether you are supported by others or not, this essence sustains you if you feel 'the odd one out'. It brings inner strength and endurance if you face opposition, obstacles or extra struggle because of your stance on life.

Self-reliance....   Stepping out on a path that is unsupported by others, you can derive benefit from the support of **Happy Wanderer** essence. This essence has an independent and individual quality that inspires you to be self-reliant and determined to do things by yourself if necessary. Overriding feelings of insecurity or apprehension, it imbues qualities of self-assurance and determination.

Inner conviction....   Ian White (ABFE) writes that '**Sturt Desert Rose** essence helps people follow their own inner convictions and morality and do what they know that they have to do. **Sturt Desert Rose** gives people the strength to be true to themselves'. This essence helps you as an individual to be true to your own path, even if it is contrary to that of the group. The other qualities that this essence instils are greater self-esteem and release of guilt or regret arising from past actions.

I can do it.... **Walnut** essence is of great benefit if you need to resist the influence or convictions of others. This essence encourages you to break through any limitations, restrictions or control from others and to pursue with faith and determination your own beliefs and goals. It endows you with the required faith and determination to pursue your objectives and in making adjustments to external changes and transitions.

> *'I believe in myself and I have the
> strength to do what is right for me'*

Balancing Aquarian energy

You are constantly busy, thinking, analyzing and planning ... but this level of mental focus can be draining and devitalizing for many Aquarians. Your independent nature can distance you from others, making you feel lonely, abandoned and dejected. It is important, however, that you put your energy into doing your own thing, even though it may be contrary to the norm, but obviously within the bounds of society.

Living too much in the mind

If you are strongly influenced by the planet Uranus, this makes you highly ingenious, original and inventive. Rather than receiving insights through your feelings and sensations, as the water signs do, your thoughts usually come to you through the concept of ideas, mental pictures or abstract images. A busy head full of churning thoughts can however deplete your life-force, making relaxation and sleeping difficult and disturbed.

Restoring.... **Nasturtium** essence restores vitality if you find that intense mental focus exhausts you. This essence grounds an individual who works predominantly in their head.

Calming....	***Yellow Boronia*** essence brings a soothing, calming influence to the dominance of mental activity, yet at the same time it fosters concentration and brings focus to scattered thoughts. Its positive qualities centre the mind so that you become capable of deep contemplation and reflection.
An open mind....	According to Ian White (ABFE), those people who need ***Yellow Cowslip Orchid*** essence 'are focused so much in the intellect that they are often blocked off from many of their feelings. When they are out of balance they have a tendency to be excessively critical and judgmental, as well as aloof, withdrawn and overly cautious about accepting things'. This essence encourages an open mind, compassion and acceptance of people and ideas, free of the tendency to pass judgment unfairly.
Focus....	If you tend to be an absent-minded Aquarian, then you can benefit from ***Sundew*** essence, which helps you to stay focused instead of mentally absent. This essence replaces feelings of disconnectedness, forgetfulness or vagueness with attention to the present. Returning you to the reality of the here and now, this essence increases concentration and purposefulness.

'My mind is balanced with feeling and emotion'

Healing feelings of separation, loneliness or isolation

Receptive....	If at times you feel lonely, isolated or rejected by other people, then ***Veronica*** essence gives you the confidence to make contact with others. It overcomes feelings of alienation, or the fear that you will always be alone, by helping you to become more receptive and open to others—and to express yourself without worry of how you will be received.
Connected....	The healing qualities of ***Single Delight*** essence bring about a state of lightness. If you feel separate or disconnected from others, this essence creates a feeling of connection with all living things. Steve Johnson writes, 'Its vibration opens our hearts and brings a remembrance of the support we have always had, helping us replace our feelings of isolation with a factual energetic experience of connectedness with life'.

Belonging....	**Tall Yellow Top** essence not only encourages self-acceptance, it also promotes a sense of belonging, helping you to feel accepted by others. Healing feelings of alienation or abandonment, it restores energy to the heart so that you feel more open and connected to others.
Comfortable with oneself....	According to Sabina Pettitt, the challenges of **Hermit Crab** essence are 'Loneliness and Avoidance'. She writes the following about this essence. 'In counterpoint to this ability to appreciate aloneness it is also an effective energy pattern to introduce when someone is always avoiding—relationships, life, moving forward'.

> *'Forming bonds and connections*
> *with others comes easily to me'*

Keeping positive and light

Inspired by inventive ideas and mental images, you can become despondent when your reforms and plans are restricted by practicalities. If Saturn, the more serious of Aquarius's two ruling planets, holds more sway over you, this can tend to make your mind rather stern, causing you to become negative in your thinking and succumbing to heaviness at times. It is important for you to think positively and to remember, 'You are what you think'.

Uplifting....	The uplifting energy of **Chiming Bells** essence is energizing and regenerating if you are sad or discouraged. It endows inner strength and hope, together with joy of life, especially if you have become out of touch with yourself. 'But most importantly, the essence of **Chiming Bells** is a vibrational bridge that helps us connect with a real and tangible source of support that is available to us at all times, no matter how lost we feel—the loving energy of the Divine Mother' (Steve Johnson).
Acceptance....	**Tall Yellow Top** essence addresses a sense of alienation, a feeling of not fitting in or belonging, which can lead to depression. If you find it difficult to relate to your emotions, thus increasing your sense of alienation, this essence helps to create a better balance of head and heart energy, enabling you to feel

more comfortable with your feelings. It increases your sense of belonging and instils feelings of acceptance so that you no longer feel alone.

Lightness....

Symbolic of the qualities that it heals, the flower **Single Delight** grows in sheltered areas away from the light and sun, with its blossom pointing towards the ground. This essence is useful if you enter a period of darkness and find it difficult to raise your head up. It heals by lifting your spirits to be aware of the light that surrounds you, and it increases awareness of your connection with all living things. This helps you feel no longer without help or out there on your own.

Hope....

The positive energy of **Scotch Broom** essence is elevating if at times you become bogged down, pessimistic or depressed, especially in relation to your role in the world or about the uncertainty of world events. In keeping with your awareness of humanity, it infuses feelings of hope, encouragement and optimism in global affairs.

> 'My thoughts are full of healing,
> vitalizing energy and light'

Finding your place and way in society

The typical Aquarian believes in equality for all, and in working together to produce something that will benefit society. Energized by the energy of a group situation, you are happy to be involved with others who share your values. However it is important for you to maintain your individuality, distinct from your position within (say) a club or community.

Express your truth....

Enhancing your individuality and uniqueness, **The Rose** essence fosters self-expression if you feel different or unusual. Loosening up any fear of exposure or revelation, it enables you to express your truth, even if this is radical or extreme. This essence is for 'those whose role challenges them to openly express the light of their truth and divinity in all areas of their life'. 'It helps us to find ways to understand what it is that we wish to express, how we can do so, and how we can integrate and develop all the necessary skills and resources, so that our vision can unfold' (Rose Titchiner).

| *Break new ground....* | The healing qualities of **Yellow Dryas** essence sustain the Aquarian who feels isolated and unsupported. Helping you find your identity and see your purpose within the larger scheme of things, it enables you to have a clear perspective of your life-experiences. Inspiring you to break new ground or lead the way, this essence brings an enlightened view of how your past experiences are valuable and relevant to your life now. |

| *Step into the unknown....* | Most appropriate for Aquarius, the key words 'Liberation and Freedom' are used by Marion Leigh to describe the healing qualities of **Hazel** essence. This essence helps to break through limiting patterns, fixed ideas and ties. Free of these impediments, you are able to tap into clear insights about your purpose in life. This essence helps you to step into the unknown, free from burdensome ways of thinking, and to have trust, faith and motivation. |

| *Connect with your purpose....* | Steve Johnson writes that the variety of **Shooting Star** (*Dodecatheon frigidum*) he uses in this Alaskan essence grows high up in the mountains, far away from humans and their habitations. These conditions link the essence aptly to the Aquarian who can feel unwanted, cut-off and distant. This essence can heal feelings of alienation, discomfort and generally not fitting in. Its welcoming energy helps you to connect with your purpose in life and to understand why you are here. |

| *Honour your truth....* | The essence **Indian Pipe** encourages you to be involved in a relationship with a group or association, yet still able to express your individuality and exclusiveness. Embodying the attributes of honour and reverence, this essence cultivates self-nurturing, self-worth and respect for others. |

> *'I am free to follow my heart and*
> *to do what is right for me'*

Relating and communicating

☞ For the Soul-lessons, see pp. 13 & 25

Involvement in relationships and working towards cooperation and harmony helps you to work upon your soul-lesson of brother/sisterhood. When mentally attuned yourself to the minds of others, you can help unite hearts and minds.

Advancing your social consciousness

After working out which of your many skills and talents can benefit society, you can then blend your individual purpose with whatever benefits the greater community.

Balancing needs....

The essence **Quaking Grass** increases your social conscience and encourages you to find your identity through associations or in group work. Most importantly, it helps you to balance your own needs with those of others.

Your place in society....

Also helping you to do your work in society, the essence **Sweet Pea** conveys a feeling of connection with humanity. Fostering a sense of attachment and commitment to your community, this essence instils within you a sense of your own special place in society, in addition to encouraging supportive relationships with others.

Sharing....

Developing and enhancing social skills, the affable qualities of **Mallow** essence promote friendly and sharing qualities. It helps you to feel self-confident and secure when involved in social situations, encouraging you to reach out to others with warmth.

Identifying with the group....

According to Marion Leigh, the essence of **Lime** helps to anchor universal love in the heart. She goes on to say that 'essence of **Lime** can empower and encourage us to work for peace and spiritual harmony on earth'. Helping to promote group consciousness in an individual, this essence resonates well with the Aquarian ability to identity with the collective rather than the individual self.

Co-operation....

The keywords for **Coral** essence are 'harmony' and 'cooperation', and the following words aptly describe this essence's link with the Aquarian's principles, 'Unity and diversity—living together in harmony. We are many and we are one' (Sabina Pettitt). This essence encourages respect for others and the skills necessary to live harmoniously in a community with others.

> *'I use my skills and talents for the greater good'*

Promoting group energy and harmony

Many Aquarians like to get involved by using the Aquarian energy to champion new causes, introduce reforms or promote brother- and sisterhood.

Creating harmony....

An important essence for Aquarians working within groups, the essence **Harvest Lily** fills you with a balanced and harmonious energy that radiates out and is felt by others. Its unifying qualities are useful in negotiation, resolution of tension and in creating harmony between opposing groups. It assists you to be appreciative of another's point of view and it enhances the skills necessary to provide support for the group, yet at the same time it enables you to express your individuality.

Common purpose....

According to Vasudeva and Kadambii Barnao, the saying for **Ursinia** essence is 'Manifesting the Collective Ideal'. They write how this essence enables an individual 'to see clearly how to tackle problems between people' and 'to accept the reality of group dynamics and retain their idealism'. The essence brings wisdom and optimism during times of discouragement or disillusionment when working with others. It encourages you to take responsibility for helping others through their individual difficulties in order that all may work in common purpose for the collective goal.

Being involved....

Assisting you to feel part of the group, **Red Feather Flower** essence boosts supportive and sharing qualities. It replaces feelings of isolation with the enthusiasm to be involved with or to share in responsibilities with either family or community life.

> *'I serve humanity by encouraging brother/sisterhood and inspiring harmony and cooperation'*

Appreciation of others' beliefs

Not easily deviating from their firm principles, typical Aquarians often assume that their ideas or knowledge are the only way, but not everyone shares their concepts. Sometimes Aquarians are incensed by injustice or overly opinionated with extreme or fanatical beliefs, something that can cause divisions between others.

Hearing others....	**Vervain** essence assists you in seeing things from a wider perspective and helps you be openminded enough not to impose your strong opinions on others. It influences you to permit others their own opinions, without feeling threatened yourself.
Tolerance....	The mature Aquarian is committed to unity and equality for all, but when out of balance this commitment can manifest as intolerance and prejudice. The essence **Slender Rice Flower** helps you to promote harmony and cooperation within yourself and in a group, by overcoming any narrow-mindedness. It helps in conflict-resolution and it is useful in overcoming the judgmental attitudes that may operate in racial issues or religious dogma. Its flexible, tolerant and cooperative qualities encourage you to work for the common good.
Under-standing, acceptance....	Ian White (ABFE) associates the essence **Yellow Cowslip Orchid** with the Aquarian's element, Air, 'for Air is very closely connected with social order, group activity and harmony'. He continues, about the positive qualities of this essence: 'an open and inquisitive mind, the ability to grasp concepts quickly, the uncritical acceptance of people and ideas, and the ability to arbitrate fairly and compassionately while considering all of the facts'.

> *'I am respectful and considerate of other's beliefs'*

Increasing emotional warmth and involvement

Your social consciousness is usually well-developed, but Aquarians can be emotionally distant and often unreliable with those closest to them. Your self-sufficiency means that you usually hate emotional demands and are unlikely to reveal your closest feelings. You are intensely independent, with a dislike of being pinned down, of others' possessiveness or any attempt to inhibit your freedom.

Opening up....	**Evening Primrose** essence encourages those of you who are remote in emotional issues or reluctant to commit yourself, to open up or to be able to form lasting relationships. This essence also helps to heal feelings of rejection or alienation from others and, in particular, inadequate mothering or nurturing.
Sensitivity....	Enhancing your capacity for intimacy, **Balsam** essence increases warmth and sensitivity not only towards others but towards

yourself. Promoting bonding and harmony in relationships, this essence fosters nurturing and tenderness towards others and in the expression of love.

With heart....   When listening to and understanding others, then like the subjects of other air signs, you operate primarily from a rational point of view, often tending to shy away from your emotions. *Tall Yellow Top* essence is a significant essence for this sense of alienation, as it reconnects the head with the heart. Helping individuals connect with each other, it permits you to communicate from a position of balanced mind and heart energy.

In touch....   If you are the absent-minded Aquarian who can be distant and rather distracted in their thoughts, the essence of *Red and Green Kangaroo Paw* brings you back into the present. This essence enables you to be more in touch with others rather than unavailable and remote; it encourages closeness. It also brings the ability to share and be involved with others, instead of opting to take your attention elsewhere.

Gentleness....   The positive qualities of *Flannel Flower* essence assist you to express open, sensitive and gentle feelings in your physical and emotional interactions with others. If you do not feel comfortable with your feelings, if you experience difficulty in communicating emotions or if you withdraw from physical closeness, this essence enhances the ability to verbalize and share feelings.

> *'I give and receive with great warmth and feeling'*

Resolving possible physical imbalances

☞ *See p. 12 on how the essences work*

Please note that throughout this book suggestions of a medical nature are not in any way claiming that the essences will cure disease, and should not be followed as a substitute to consulting a qualified medical practitioner.

Blood Circulation

In addition to healing emotional wounds and restoring loving feelings, the essence *Fireweed* (PAC) improves circulation

(Sabina Pettitt). *Bluebell* (AB) essence balances energy in the heart both emotionally and physically, and is said to have a sphere of action in the veins as well as the heart (ABFH). Another Australian Bush essence, *Tall Mulla Mulla*, aids circulation disorders and also benefits problems with blood-flow to the extremities. It is advisable for conditions such as cold hands and feet, varicose veins and alopaecia.

In addition to the gem essence *Gold* as a heart healer, *Rose Quartz* and *Ruby* work at the heart level to heal emotional hurts, thus helping with circulatory difficulties. In addition to attracting fulfilling personal relationships and enhancing compassion, the essence *Foxglove* (PF) is indicated when the heart beats out of control or poor circulation is detected.

The nervous system

According to Judy Griffin (FTH), '*Ranunculus* essence assists the body to balance the energy from the central nervous system to the brain'. She writes that 'imbalanced energy in the brain can manifest in many ways, such as muscle spasms, temperamental and emotional outbursts, and chemical imbalances'.

Sabina Pettitt recommends both *Coral* and *Sea Horse* essences for the nervous system. She writes that *Coral* essence affects physical growth and mental potential, and recommends it as a very potent remedy, for the brain as well as the central nervous system.

Promoting the Aquarian principle of individuality, the energy of *Sea Horse* essence encourages you to be yourself and to express your unique talents and potential without being conditioned by what you feel you ought to be. Energizing the spine and the nervous system, it benefits any imbalances between the brain and either motor of sensory function. The vibrant and glowing energy of *Wild Pansy* essence energizes, if you feel confused, distracted, nervous or anxious. It also assists poor circulation and disturbed energy-currents, spasms and tensions in the body.

Comfrey (FES) essence is a powerful tonic for the nervous system, releasing tensions and calming stressful minds.

Psychological states associated with stress upon the nervous system can be eased with *Silver* essence. Working at a mental level, this essence releases stress on both the emotional and mental levels.

12. THE PISCES OUTLOOK ON LIFE AND HEALTH

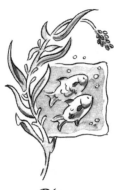

Pisces

February 19–
March 21

Quality & element:
Mutable water

Rulers:
Neptune & Jupiter

Opposite sign: Virgo

Soul-lesson: Peace

CONSTITUTION

HIGHLY impressionable, compassionate and receptive—these are the qualities that characterize the kindly Piscean, probably the least understood sign of the zodiac. The typical Pisces is ethereal, difficult to get hold of, hard to categorize. Like the subjects of other water signs, Pisceans are very responsive to the feelings and thoughts of others. Easily absorbing another's energies, it can be difficult for a Piscean to know where they end and another being starts. Merging so easily with others, they often identify more with the collective, rather than seeking out an individual identity of their own. Their self-worth often comes from service to others and this is where the gentler Piscean can be taken advantage of, sometimes over-keen to surrender his or her own needs to those of others. Creating and maintaining their own strong boundaries so that others do not adversely infiltrate their world is not only healthy but a must for Pisces if he–she is to preserve a sense of wellbeing.

Implications for health

The mystical Piscean seeks transcendence, longs to go beyond what is permanent and real. Even the more down-to-earth type would rather escape at times and in some way from reality or the harshness of the real world. Sensitive Pisceans may have difficulty in coping with the everyday world, and they need to take care, as this sign is the most likely to become dependent on drugs or drink in order to cope.

Usually highly emotional, often thinking with their hearts, they can get into situations that they do not necessarily want or need, which can be draining. They are easily overcome by any distress and upset around them, and this can drag them down and rob them of vitality.

It seems significant that in the same way that Pisceans are emotionally open and vulnerable, their bodies too are often unprotected and can become invaded by toxins and viruses, which may result in swollen or sluggish glands. Pisces rules the mucous secretions, lymph system and the fluids in the body, so these people can be prone to blood disorders, anaemia and weak immune systems.

Debbie Shapiro associates vulnerability with the emotions. She writes that emotional overload or a desire to withdraw from our feelings can affect the condition of the blood.

It is ironic that it is the feet that can give Pisceans problems, given how often they have their heads in the clouds, not wanting to come down to earth! Pisces rules the feet, and this serves as a constant reminder to them, bringing them back to earth and back in touch with the ground. As we are unable to proceed without firm steady feet to support our actions, it is crucial that Pisceans feel secure, supported, grounded and connected to the earth.

HEALING AND SELF-DEVELOPMENT FOR PISCEANS

The mind

If you are a typical Piscean, you are sensitive but often anxious because you find it difficult to cope with stress. Alternatively, your empathy for life may have drawn you into a situation that is not advantageous. Characteristically, you have no desire to be involved in conflict or turmoil, usually preferring to work quietly in the background, rather than organizing and directing others. On these occasions you tend to withdraw in order to find peace. Wellbeing for you is best maintained by making time for periods of solitude, where you are able to retreat into your own dream world and have a brief respite from everyday worries and cares. This is where you can cleanse yourself from the energies of others, to whom you are so responsive. With an ability to lose yourself in another world, you are of the sign that probably lends itself most easily to the practice of meditation—for you are usually very good at visualization or transferring yourself mentally into a tranquil and peaceful setting. This gives you the chance to withdraw temporarily and safely from everyday pressures. Your responsiveness to suggestion can also make you an ideal candidate for hypnotherapy, used in a therapeutic manner.

The body

Read the Virgo chapter too—your opposite sign.

You should always make a point of looking after your feet and investing in decent shoes. Reflexology is a treatment to which Pisceans are very responsive, and some Pisceans will even pursue this therapy as a vocation. It treats illness through pressure to areas of the feet where bodily organs and parts of the body are represented. It is interesting that through Pisces, the most mystical sign of the zodiac, a nonphysical connection is made, linking the physical body through use of pressure to the feet. It is an ideal treatment for you, as is lymphatic massage.

As the Piscean body is most often fighting bacteria internally, you have to create for yourself, too, on an outer level, a layer of protection and strength, where you can defend yourself from harmful outside influences. You need to protect yourself from being used, taken over by others or dominated by the sometimes unpleasant and hard realities of life. It is beneficial if you are able to create a secure self-image, and not rely on escapism or using dependencies of any kind as a form of avoidance. A harmless pursuit that affords a sense of escape from real life and where you can find great pleasure is some aspect of the theatrical arts. In amateur dramatics or as a spectator, you can retreat from the everyday world into a fantasy one, or actually become someone else temporarily. Television or cinema can take you safely out of yourself where you can indulge your sense of fiction and illusion. Dancing, music, poetry or art probably also appeal to you.

The spirit

USING YOUR INNER POWER AND FINDING YOUR SPIRITUAL MISSION

It is your ability unconsciously to perceive things from a non-rational viewpoint that gives you, along with the other water signs, the ability to be in touch with your intuition. In achieving your soul-lesson of inner peace, your objective is to learn to use this faculty wisely. By listening to your whispers, yet applying some wisdom and discrimination, you will not be overcome by feelings, emotions or fears. If you ignore or lose sight of your intuitive abilities, you may lose an important aspect of your being and become disconnected from your path. If things do not feel comfortable for you, then learn to listen to yourself. You can regain your inner power by connecting with your inner being and following your intuition; that inner truth will guide you and not let you down.

☞ For the Soul-lessons, see pp. 13 & 25

It is quite likely that you will want to spend some of your life serving and caring for others in some way and it is in this capacity you are often draw to charity work or improving the lot of humanity. It is most important that you develop the strength to cope with these demands by creating your own boundaries, and by putting yourself first at times.

SUGGESTED ESSENCES FOR PISCEANS

Resolving possible personality imbalances

Your approach to life is gentle and peaceful, yet the typical Piscean reluctance to face confrontation or disagreement means that life can often present you with difficulties and challenges that you cannot avoid. It is to your benefit to develop strategies to help you deal with life, and to make sure you are grounded and seeing things clearly.

Helping the sensitive Piscean cope with life

Resilience....

Cattail Pollen essence instils resilience, so that you are not weakened by difficulties in life or by shocks or upsets that you may have experienced. This essence is revitalizing and stabilizing, enabling you to stand tall and to be empowered. '**Cattail Pollen** can make it easier by helping us to strongly project our true selves out into the world so we can attract people that resonate with us at that level' (Steve Johnson).

Getting organized....

If you are the 'go with the flow' type of Piscean, you may opt out and live in disorder and chaos rather than face up to situations or circumstances. A potent essence that deals with these disorganized or muddled states is **Disciple of the Heart**. It helps teach you to structure and organize yourself and your life, so you understand how to create flexible patterns of working and being that are personal and meaningful, in addition to inspiring you to fulfill your true potential.

Stability....

If it is difficult for you to find emotional stability when surrounded by discord, then the essence **Rose Cone Flower** can help provide a safe inner space, where disturbed and edgy feelings give way to ease and calm. This essence enables you to find a peaceful place within, without having to have your external surroundings and circumstances just right.

> *'I am strong and empowered and I deal with whatever comes into my life realistically'*

Seeing and thinking with clarity

If there are times when you do not face up to yourself or situations, you can become confused, lost in your thoughts, or even deceived. Not wanting to see things as they really are can result in muddled and dreamy states.

Focused....

The grounding qualities of **Sundew** essence clear vagueness and help you pay attention to details and be decisive. They enable you to stay focused in the present, without the tendency to drift off or withdraw mentally or physically. This essence helps you to ground your ideas, visions and imaginations and inspires you to find ways of relating them to the material world.

Illumination.... Shattering your illusions and helping you to see with clarity, the essence **Bladderwort** deals with confusion and uncertainty. If you need to improve your abilities of discrimination to avoid being taken advantage of or deceived, this essence increases your inner knowing, so the truth of a situation or a circumstance becomes clearly illuminated.

Concentration.... For the dreamy Piscean who finds it easy to drift off and forget what they had intended to achieve, the essence **Pink Trumpet Flower** can assist. It helps to consolidate vague or unconnected thoughts and it promotes clarity and purpose in order to realize your objectives. Encouraging inner strength, the essence has the ability to eliminate distractions and to maintain your thinking in a very direct manner, so that your mind does not wander or lose its concentration until the job is complete.

Clarity.... The key words for **Brown Kelp** essence are 'Clarity' and 'Freedom'. This essence inspires you to be able to find what you are looking for within. Helping you to separate yourself from a head full of busy thoughts, it enables you to feel more comfortable with any observations that may arise and to trust in the flow of life rather than hold on to old survival patterns. Sabina Pettitt writes that the type of person that can benefit from this essence is the type who 'tends to get in their own way through fear and confusion'.

> *'I see and think with clarity'*

Coping with avoidance

As Pisces is a mutable sign, you are adaptable and flexible, but your desire for freedom means that you usually prefer not to commit yourself too much. Evasive, unavailable or inclined to run away, the elusive Piscean can slip through the net just when it is time to make a commitment or a decision or to deal with a difficulty!

Reliable....	The essence **Many-Headed Dryandra** brings the maturity necessary to commit to others or to an area of life that requires consistency or dedication. If you become overwhelmed, cannot cope or feel that everything is too much for you, then this essence unites fulfilment with dependability. It encourages you to find pleasure from being stable and reliable in life.
Good judgment....	**Wattle** essence has a mature energy, ensuring that you become aware of reality and face up to situations. Instead of your opting out of important issues and not dealing with problems, this essence helps impart understanding of the consequences of your actions. It instils alertness, awareness and the wisdom to discern good judgment in all of your choices. Not surprisingly the saying for this essence is 'Worldly Wise' (Barnao).
Live in the present....	The flower essence **Clematis** addresses inattention, indifference and confused states. If you are an unrealistic or idealistic Piscean, this essence assists you in utilizing your colourful imagination and making workable your creative or artistic abilities. It makes it easier for you to live in the present and to handle any unpleasant situations that may arise without escaping to a fantasy world.
Facing up to issues....	In addition to helping you cope with a lack of endurance, **Coconut** essence enables you to deal with concerns, without avoiding them. This essence imparts a realistic energy that helps you face up to issues or difficulties with realism, and the determination to complete tasks with commitment.

> *'I am realistic and face up to life'*

Staying grounded

Elsewhere in his or her thoughts, or overwhelmed by the pressure and hassle of living, the extremely sensitive and dreamy Piscean can resort to living in his or her own world, removed from reality.

The real world....	**Fawn Lily** essence fosters acknowledgment of the real world and the strength to become involved and to manage everyday matters. Those who need it 'are naturally inclined to states of

contemplation, meditation and prayer. It is easier for them to stay in these modes of spirituality, rather than to be involved with the world'. 'Such persons need to disseminate the great gifts which have accumulated in their beings in order to evolve and progress' (Kaminski and Katz). This essence also stimulates natural healing capabilities and encourages an individual to share and utilize their spiritual gifts and skills with others.

Courage....

If you are a spiritually-minded Piscean who finds it difficult to stay on this planet, then **Stitchwort** essence is grounding and helps you to feel safe and secure. Enabling sensitive souls to see through the illusion of fear, it provides the courage to forge ahead and break new ground. This essence assures you that you are not alone and will always be sustained with divine support through your life-experience.

Unite....

In addition to allaying unknown fears, the essence **West Australian Smokebush** reinforces your strong, grounded connection. It unites the body and mind, restoring clear-headedness if you feel vague, disconnected or directionless. This essence is strengthening after stress and trauma, as it reintegrates the levels of your being that may have become split or disorientated.

Resistance....

The healing qualities of **Rainbow Glacier** essence help the individual who is more focused in the heavenly realms than the earthly dimensions. Steve Johnson prepared this Alaskan environmental essence from water taken at the terminus of Rainbow Glacier, high in the Alaskan Range in the eastern part of the state. 'This essence also works to alleviate deep levels of resistance to being present in one's body, resistance that is often the result of an extremely painful experience' (Steve Johnson).

> *'I am down-to-earth and live in the real world'*

Inner guidance

You can benefit from keeping in touch with your inner guidance and intuition, but if you are anxious about occult matters, this fear can block you from approaching anything on a spiritual level. As you tend to function mainly on an intuitive level, ignoring your inner impressions is not advantageous and can give you doubts and worries which demoralize you.

Trust....

Helping you to become more in touch with your intuition and impressions, to trust in your inner feelings and express yourself with more insight from your intuition: this is the essence **Bush Fuchsia**.

The answer is within....

Angelsword essence works primarily at a subtle level, cutting through spiritual confusion, establishing clear communication with your higher self and helping you receive spiritual truths. It is appropriate whatever way you receive your messages from within, whether through intuition, books, teachings or meditation. It has a protective quality, clearing negative influences, eliminating uncertainty and enabling you to find wisdom.

Awareness....

Mint Bush essence not only provides you with the ability to cope at difficult and testing times, but it also fosters an awareness of spirituality and helps it emerge during these stressful times. This essence makes it easier for you to view restrictions and limitations in your life as an opportunity to make progress on a deeper inner level. **Mint Bush** also provides support at the times your values are shifting and the structure of your life seems to be crumbling and falling away.

Higher guidance....

If you are spiritually aware, but hesitant to manifest your true identity in the World, then the essence **Icelandic Poppy** enables you to shine as your divine self. This essence can be used to re-establish a link to your higher guidance if the challenges of life have left you feeling out of touch with spiritual wisdom or awareness. The affirmation for this essence is: 'I am a radiant spiritual being. My spiritual power constantly shines outward into all aspects of my life' (Steve Johnson).

> *'I trust my intuition and perceptions'*

Balancing Piscean energy

You may be keenly aware of the non-real world, highly impressionable, sensitive and perceptive to everything happening around you, but your Piscean imagination can get the better of you. Subject to all sorts of worries, you may end up distressed and exhausted and with your vitality drained. Learning to remain at peace and to strengthen your personal boundaries will provide protection and enable you to become stronger.

Overcoming panic, terror and fear

Succumbing to the workings of your wild imagination, your thoughts and your perceptions, you can become fearful of just about anything! Vague fears seem to arise from nowhere; this uneasiness can make you apprehensive and fearful about life.

Feeling safe.... Aspen essence dispels these feelings of nervousness and unease, enabling you to feel safe and secure enough to tackle life without fear. It brings a sense of security and enables you to trust that you are safe and protected.

Strength.... You can be drained and immobilized when nervousness and anxiety give way to extreme terror or panic. *Rock Rose* essence deals with these overwhelming situations if you feel helpless or unable to cope, by gathering your forces together and restabilizing you. Restoring courage and bravery, it enables you to deal with situations with unwavering, steady strength. It is also one of the constituents of *Rescue Remedy*, a combination of five different essences that can be used to bring calmness during nightmares, after accidents and in emergency situations. When produced by the Healing Herbs Company, this Bach essence is known as *Five Flower Remedy*.

Conquering fear.... The saying for *Ribbon Pea* essence is 'Safe within the universe' (Barnao). Feelings of fear, apprehension, anxiety and foreboding are quelled by this essence as it helps liberate you from deep dread or terror. Its positive energy is calming and composing so you can conquer any indefinable worries and go forward in life with serenity.

'I have no reason to fear; I am always safe'

Support for the vulnerable Piscean

Although gentle and caring, you can be too open and vulnerable to life or to others. Even if you are a Piscean who puts on a hard outer shell around themselves, you probably have an exposed side, which you are usually trying to protect.

Deter-
mination....

If you feel vulnerable to suffering, naïve or just unable to cope with the harsh realities of life, the essence of **Swan River Myrtle** can provide you with inner strength. This essence supplies the necessary determination to walk away from situations or people that are unjust or unreasonable, or the awareness not to put yourself into situations in which you are compromised or taken for granted. Either way, it provides insights into unfairness or injustice, whether you are the victim or the perpetrator.

Optimism....

When you have either been through tough times or experienced trauma and sadness, the regenerating quality of **Giving Hands** essence helps to restore your optimism and hope. Your giving nature can easily be exploited or mistreated, leaving you feeling crushed, abused and wanting to withdraw from life. This essence helps to heal this heaviness and to bring back a joy for living and interaction with others.

True to
yourself....

The cleansing attributes of **Antiseptic Bush** essence are 'internal integrity' and 'being true to one's inner light'. (Barnao) This essence is ideal if you find you are too open to the influence of others or if you are frustrated at getting yourself into situations where you feel compromised.

> *'Whatever life throws my way, I feel supported and able to cope'*

Maintaining peace at all costs

You are inclined to pick up a plethora of feelings and emotions from others or from the environment, which can leave you feeling 'adrift on a choppy sea'. Your erratic and fluctuating emotions can cause you great anguish and torment. The following suggested essences help the sensitive soul to maintain a sense of stability and composure.

Calm....

The watery association of the gem essence, **Aquamarine**, links well with the aquatic Pisces. **Aquamarine** helps to calm Piscean nerves, balance emotions and reduce fears and worries. Helpful if you feel a sense of disorientation or not being 'present', this essence creates a serene, centred and ordered state of mind.

Peace....

Red Clover essence deals with the panic and terror that can sometimes overtake you. When you are fearful and anxious, this essence assists you establish peace and stability in your life. It helps you to feel that you are safe in your own space and to recognize that fear is an illusion.

Relaxed....

Scottish Primrose essence develops inner peace and stillness where worry, nervousness or anxieties exist. In coping with panic, trauma or shock, this essence helps bring a sense of grounding to extreme, overwhelming situations, which can result in you feeling 'out of your body'. It harmonizes and re-stores natural rhythms so you can feel back 'in sync', relaxed, with all parts of your being in balance in another. If you are brokenhearted, anguished, or tackling conflict or crisis, this essence is soothing; it reinstates peace and tranquillity in the heart and instils courage and harmony.

> *'I am composed, calm and at peace'*

Safe spirituality

As a natural psychic, you absorb feelings and sense things that other people are not aware of. However, these highly-tuned perceptions can make you nervous and apprehensive.

Overwhelmed....

Lavender essence is effective if you are highly absorbent of spiritual influences and the toll this takes on you overwhelms you physically and emotionally. This essence restores emotional balance and helps you moderate your sensitivity to psychic energy and the strain this puts on you physically. This essence is soothing, calming and balancing whether it is a feeling of depleted energy, nervousness or sleeplessness that you suffer.

Too open....

Being receptive to sensations that are beyond your normal senses can make you very vulnerable and cause you to worry unnecessarily. The supportive essence **Purple Monkeyflower** instils calm when you are frightened or overwhelmed by any aspect of the occult. Establishing a love-based approach to spiritual experience, this essence motivates you to trust in your own spirituality, instead or feeling alarm or trepidation in such matters.

Feeling threatened....

In addition to protecting against those who may drain your energy, **Fringed Violet** essence protects against spiritual attack. **Grey Spider Flower** essence can be relied on to implant courage and calmness during intense fear or in any situation where you experience panic and terror. Ian White (ABFE) writes that '**Grey Spider Flower** can be used with **Fringed Violet** for protection against psychic attacks, or at times when you feel your life is threatened. These remedies will help to develop trust and faith and the knowledge that the Light can always be called on to protect you'.

Unknown territory....

The challenge of **Urchin** essence is 'Fear of the unknown' (Sabina Pettitt). Surrounded by protective, spiky, purple quills, the energy of this sea creature supplies you with a safe sanctuary within. This essence provides emotional shelter and protection whenever you are exploring unknown territory of a spiritual nature. It also provides safety from psychic assault and is helpful in alleviating worry, obsessions and addictions.

A universal perspective....

The aquamarine nature of **White Nymph Waterlily (Miani)** essence resonates well with watery Pisces. Settling the emotions and inducing inner calm, this essence encourages you to integrate a spiritual viewpoint, especially during difficult or frustrating times. 'The essence of tranquillity that encourages pulling back the layers to reach the Soul level. To inspire using the higher self to integrate and respond to Life from the most Universal perspective possible for one's evolution at the time, rather than one's personal perspective' (Barnao).

> *'Protective golden light surrounds*
> *me and keeps me calm and safe'*

Dealing with addictions and dependencies

Seeing the world through rose-coloured glasses is the preference of some Pisceans, as opposed to coping with the prob-

lems and the practicalities of everyday life. Sometimes this means dependence on stimulants such as drugs, alcohol or other excesses in order to avoid reality or bring you relief or freedom from the cruelness of the world.

Self-reliance.... **Milkweed** essence imparts the strength and self-reliance to cope with any dependencies. It instils independence, restores self-awareness and brings a healthy sense of ego, so you are able to manage the demands and responsibilities of normal life.

Willpower.... Breaking the hold that old habits may have on you, including addictions, dependencies and obsessions, **Blue China Orchid** essence takes on any such destructive behaviour-patterns. It increases willpower and self-control, enabling you to have the strength and discipline to break the mould, restore wholeness and embark on new experiences.

Motivation.... Sabina Pettitt's affirmation for **Forsythia** essence is, 'I am willing to change. I have the inner resources and energy required to change'. Working on unhelpful patterns of behaviour, habits or addictions, this essence provides the motivation, power and willingness to break and conquer alcohol, drug, tobacco or similar addictions. It helps to move one on from unhealthy relationships or thought-patterns that hinder or hold one back.

Regular patterns.... Important in giving up addictions, and dealing with cravings, the essence **Morning Glory** not only helps break addictive patterns, but removes the associated side effects and re-establishes a regular pattern and stability in your life.

> *'I am strong and depend only on myself'*

Relating and communicating

Your kindly nature often finds you in 'people' professions. If you are drawn to serve humankind through charity and volunteer roles, you need strong boundaries and you need to employ good protective techniques. Becoming less influenced by unseen fears and less vulnerable to the energies of others will enable you to give better service to others without compromising yourself.

Standing true to yourself

With a tendency to give away too much of yourself to others, it is essential you establish balance in relationships, especially those involving 'caring', otherwise you can suffer.

Wisdom....

Leafless Orchid essence focuses on deepening your understanding of exactly what caring for others is. Its supportive energy increases wisdom, so that you know exactly when to stand back and exactly how much is healthy to give to others. This essence is excellent when as a carer or volunteer you become burnt out, drained or overwhelmed.

Inspire....

If your sensitivity and humanitarian disposition mean that you are overwhelmed witnessing suffering and injustice, then **White Spider Orchid** essence can provide support. Instead of your becoming weighed down with helplessness, this essence enthuses you to rise above any unfairness and misery. Known as 'The Care Giver', it is 'to inspire those in the caring professions and in volunteer service, engendering a higher perspective on the purpose of this pain in the journey of the soul' (Barnao).

Rejuvenate....

Working at both the emotional and mental level, the energy of **Alpine Mint Bush** essence has a renewing quality, revitalizing individuals worn down by responsibility for others. If you work in any sort of caring position or in the service or welfare of others, this essence rejuvenates and increases motivation and enthusiasm in your work.

> *'Standing true in all my relationships, I give what I can without jeopardizing my own wellbeing'*

Providing protection from the energies of others

So good at picking up other's feelings and moods, you can usually sense what another feels, or the dynamics of a situation, without a verbal explanation.

Staying intact....

If you easily take on the feelings or absorb the energies of others, you can benefit from **Fringed Violet** essence. The qualities of this essence provide protection from the negative and draining energies of other people. Helping to keep the life-force intact and balanced, it can also be taken after shock, trauma or surgery.

Shielding.... The shielding power of **Hybrid Pink Fairy Cowslip Orchid** essence creates a well of inner strength and resilience. This essence helps you become less affected by the emotions of others and able to respond sensitively rather than reacting emotionally.

Protecting.... **Guardian,** a combination of several Alaskan flower essences, is extremely useful for all sensitive people. It protects by surrounding you with a strong energetic boundary, preventing the absorption of unwanted energies. Defended and protected, you can feel safe and guarded in your own space with this essence.

Centering.... Very appropriate to the Piscean psyche, **Daisy** essence assists the sensitive and vulnerable Piscean by creating an energetic barrier that is impervious to any confusion, disorder or distraction. Protecting and centering, this essence shields from overwhelming situations and helps you to stay focused on your purpose. It is strengthening if you are the oversensitive type or easily influenced against your better judgment.

> *'I am totally protected and remain unaffected by disharmonious energies'*

Creating strong boundaries

A safe place.... If you feel like withdrawing or cutting yourself off from others because you are so overwhelmed, the essence **Monkshood** helps you to define strong boundaries. Its protective quality assists you to overcome fearfulness and enables you to feel that you are in a safe place, without actually having to withdraw physically.

Attract the right people.... **One-Sided Wintergreen** essence assists if you find yourself involved with people or situations that are not to your advantage. This essence not only deepens your understanding of how your energy can affect others, but it also helps you to give out the type of energy that draws towards you only those that support your highest good. It enables you still to care deeply for others, but only where you are appreciated and not taken advantage of.

Conviction....

It is easy for you to lose sight of your own goals and objectives when you concentrate too much on attending others or serving an ideal or vision. ***Centaury*** essence fosters wisdom, so awareness of your own individuality and convictions is strong and firm. Creating a better balance between others' needs and your own, it enables you not to lose sight of your own mission in life.

> *'I appreciate myself and I am*
> *strong in my own convictions'*

Avoiding the victim or martyr role

The vulnerable Piscean can be drawn into situations that are not always advantageous to him or her. It is usually your first instinct to show compassion and to help another, but you can end up being taken advantage of, exploited or suffering in some way. You can also find it extremely difficult to extricate yourself from a situation, even when you know you are being used. Feeling hard done-by, you can take on the victim role at times.

Self-worth....

Ensuring that you are not exploited by others, the essence of **Urchin Dryandra** increases self appreciation and boosts self-respect. This new-found self-worth prompts changes in the dynamics of relationships, thus ensuring that your future relationships are built on healthy foundations. Moving you out of a victim role, this essence releases sadness, hurt, inferiority or feelings of being unappreciated, replacing them with positive feelings about yourself.

Personal power....

The essence of **Southern Cross** fosters awareness that we each create our own reality by the way we think and act. Therefore the more optimistic we are, the more we draw positive people and circumstances towards us. The reverse of this thinking is creating a victim-consciousness, where by continually affirming negativity and pessimism we become stuck in this mentality and all that it attracts. **Southern Cross** essence implants the message that the universe always gives you exactly what you expect; so if you continually expect life to be affirmative, abundant and joyous, then this is the sort of energy that you draw towards yourself. The supporting and encouraging energy of this essence has the same effect as increasing your personal power through positive thinking. It pulls you out of victim mentality by instilling responsibility for all your actions.

Self-assured.... Increasing inner strength is one of the attributes of **Geraldton Wax** essence. It improves self-assurance, so you find that you are able to stand your own two feet without being easily influenced, pressured or compromised by others. Neither do you bow down or give in except to what you feel to be right.

Discrimination.... If your natural ability to minister to others becomes unbalanced, you can easily be exploited, sometimes to the point of being abused. **Centaury** essence gives you the power to be your own person and to follow your own inner mission, while still giving service to others in a balanced manner. It encourages your powers of discrimination, allowing you to say 'no' when necessary.

> *'I am self-assured and powerful and*
> *I hold myself in great respect'*

Resolving possible physical imbalances

☛ *See p. 12 on how the essences work*

Please note that throughout this book suggestions of a medical nature are not in any way claiming that the essences will cure disease, and should not be followed as a substitute to consulting a qualified medical practitioner.

The blood system

Louse Hay writes the following about anaemia, 'The heart, of course, represents love, while our blood represents joy. Our hearts lovingly pump joy throughout our bodies. When we deny ourselves joy and love, the heart shrivels and becomes cold. As a result, the blood gets sluggish and we creep our way to anaemia, angina, and heart attacks'.

The essence **Bluebell** (AB) helps to open the heart, and in doing so assists in dealing with blood disorders such as anaemia. **Rose Quartz** gem essence also operates at the heart level, healing emotional hurts, increasing self-love and impacting physically upon the blood and on circulatory difficulties. Stimulating the life-force, *Kapok Bush* essence motivates you to respond to life with willingness. It boosts vitality and works on conditions such as anaemia or low blood pressure. For the individual who is anaemic and withdrawn, the essence *Dianthus* enhances self-worth, incites passion for life and encourages release of anger if it has been channelled into apathy rather than released.

The lymph and immune systems

In order for the immune system to be functioning at its full potential, the lymph system needs to be efficient at removing toxins and dead bacteria from the body's tissues. Ian White (ABFH) recommends *Bush Iris* essence to treat 'the following types of symptoms which all stem from a sluggish lymphatic system: oedema, elephantiasis, acne, eczema and other skin rashes; body odour; and chronic illnesses generally' .

Judy Griffin's 'Petite Fleur' range of flower essences contains several essences that assist the immune system when it is in a weakened state and aid the lymph system to battle against viruses. Supporting the body in detoxifying fatty deposits and unclogging the lymph system are the essences *Soapwort, Aquilegia Columbine* and *Red Carnation*.

The 'fighter' essences include *Silver Lace*, which works with the body's ability to synthesize interferon, a protein that inhibits viral attack; *Snapdragon,* which raises the consciousness of the immune system and *Lily* which prevents anxiety and worry breaking down the immune system. In the same way that *Gaillardia* essence supports an individual to overcome opposition and difficulties, it works with macrophages in the immune system, whose job it is to intercept and conquer foreign substances. A combination of the above essences produces a powerful defensive mix for the immune system, to which you may add others if required to promote drainage for a sluggish lymph system.

EPILOGUE:
THE ESSENCE OF
MASTERING OUR LIVES

THROUGHOUT our lifetimes we are presented with many challenges and obstacles to overcome, which inevitably force us to learn on some level. We are also afforded opportunities that provide just the right occasions and situations for our growth and self-development. While they may not necessarily be seen as such at the time, difficulties and tests can be viewed in the same light as opportunities, although a longterm outlook (usually in retrospect) is often required into how events may have shaped our lives and accelerated our progression on a personal level. How we handle our trials in life matters greatly, as our response shapes the way things develop for us in the future. Our type of personality enables us to cope with grace and understanding, or with awkwardness and upset, the later of which may cause mental or emotional, perhaps even physical discomfort.

As we have seen from the previous chapters, we have aids to call to our assistance. Greater self-knowledge through astrology helps reassure us about who think we are and who we are capable of being, but also warns us where weaknesses may lie. Aligning ourselves with an individual spiritual mission clarifies direction toward a path or course in life. Equipped with our own personalized portfolio of essences, we have a tool kit to assist us on our life's journey. Expanding our awareness with flower essences, we realize that the world is not conspiring against us, but offering us continual opportunities for self-development. In time, with the essences' support, we can become more able to steer our own ship through life, and with maturity and wisdom, regardless of whether life at certain points pounds us against the rocks or plunges us to the depths.

Ultimately, as master of our own lives, rather than slaves, we may find we experience fewer of these events, by recognizing of what they are teaching us. As we become less driven by the lower aspects of our natures, we grow increasingly able to direct our will and emotions in more productive ways. Eventually transcending the qualities of our individual horoscopes and incorporating the best of all the zodiac signs, we attain our highest potential—emotionally, mentally, physically and spiritually.

Obviously, our behaviour and thinking can have a profound influence on those around us. This is especially so for the parents among us, who have a huge responsibility in influencing a new generation.* Regardless of who we are or what our role is, we are accountable first to ourselves, and this means endeavouring to become the finest models we can be. Through creating the best possible circumstances (emotionally, mentally, physically and spiritually) for ourselves we not only benefit, but we shall be favourably affecting others, including our children. This is instrumental in raising the consciousness of everyone. The sooner we start the better!

*See page 270, about the 'Purely Essences' range.

APPENDICES

1. BIBLIOGRAPHY AND READING LIST

BARNAO, Vasudeva and Kadambii, *Australian Flower Essences for the Twenty-first Century*. Australia (Australian Flower Essence Academy) 1997.

BARNARD, Julian and Martine, *The Healing Herbs of Edward Bach*. London (Ashgrove Publishing), 1995.

DEVI, Lila, *The Essential Flower Essence Handbook*. USA (Hay House), 1998.

EMOTO, Masuru, *Messages from Water* (two volumes). Japan (Hado Kyoikusha Co Ltd), 2002

GERBER, Richard, M.D., *Vibrational Medicine*. USA (Bear & Co), 1996.

GRIFFIN, Judy, *Flowers that Heal* (FTH in text). New York, NY (Paraview Press), 2002.

GRIFFIN, Judy, Ph D, *The Healing Flowers* (THF in text).Texas (Herbal Health Inc.Publication), 2000

HARVEY, Clare G., *The New Encyclopaedia of Flower Remedies*. London (Watkins Publishing), 2007.

HAY, Louise L, *You Can Heal Your Life*. London (Eden Grove Editions), 1988.

HODGSON, Joan, *Wisdom in the Stars*. Liss, Hampshire (White Eagle Publishing Trust), fourth edition, 2004.

HODGSON, Joan, *Astrology the Sacred Science*. Liss, Hampshire (White Eagle Publishing Trust), 1978

JOHNSON, Steve, *The Essence of Healing*. Alaska (Alaskan Flower Essence Project), 2000.

KAMINSKI, Patricia and KATZ, Richard, *Flower Essence Repertory*. California (The Flower Essence Society), 1994.

LEIGH, Marion, *Findhorn Flower Essences*. Findhorn, Morays (Findhorn Press), 1998

PAGE, Dr Christine R, *Frontiers of Health*. Saffron Walden (C.W. Daniel Company), 1994

PERT, Candace, *Molecules of Emotion*. UK (Simon & Schuster UK), 1998.

PETTITT, Sabina, *Energy Medicine*. Canada (Pacific Essences), 1999.

SHAPIRO, Debbie, *The Bodymind Workbook*. UK (Element Books), 1994.

TITCHINER, Rose, *Truly Divine*. Halesworth, Suffolk (Waterlily Books), 2004.

WHITE, Ian, *Australian Bush Flower Essences* (ABFE in text). Findhorn, Morays (Findhorn Press), 1998.

WHITE, Ian, *Australian Bush Flower Healing* (ABFH in text). Australia (Bantam Books), 1999.

WRIGHT, Machaelle Small, *Flower Essences*. Warrenton, VA, USA (Perelandra Ltd), 1988.

2. THE 'PURELY ESSENCES' RANGE

Addressing what is probably the most crucially influential stage of our development, the MOTHER & BABY range from Purely Essences (www.purelyessences.com) was produced specifically for parents to be, parents (or carers), babies and small children. These essences were created by myself and Shelley Sishton, to support the journey from pre-conception through pregnancy, birth and into family life together. The inspiration to produce these essences was motivated not only to address the needs of the children born nowadays, but for the well-being and benefit of the whole family unit, which in today's society is fragmented and often dysfunctional.

Conception and prenatal

PREGNANCY PARTNER
Clears cluttered emotional energies from the womb to create a joyful and sacred space for conception and for baby to grow within. This essence unites mother and baby in true partnership, preparing both for birth and beyond.

Childbirth

BIRTHING COMPANION
Offering an invitation to relax into the innate wisdom of her body during birth, this essence supports a mother through what can be an intense physical and emotional experience.

Postnatal

NURSING MOTHER
Assisting all mothers, not just those who wish to breast feed. This essence inspires a relaxed, yet confident approach to feeding. Strengthening the bond between them, it helps mothers to feel calm and assured when handling their baby.

SOOTHE BABY BLUES
The period following birth can be a vulnerable time for parents. This essence restores emotional balance and encourages self-nurturing qualities, enabling mum or dad to manage the daily demands of family life without feeling overwhelmed.

Parenting

HELLO DAD
It is not always easy to make the transition into the role of Dad especially if one is carrying preconceived ideas or expectations. This essence helps men adjust to such a major life change with an open heart and mind.

MUM'S EVERYWHERE
To help mums at any time of her life, to honour herself and to balance her own time and space with the needs of her family. It helps her maintain a healthy balance of giving and receiving.

Baby and children

WELCOME BABY
This essence, available as bath drops or room spritz, provides souls with the best possibly start. Invoking a sense of peace and reassurance, it invites baby to feel welcome and much loved here on earth.

SIBLING SUPPORT
Helps siblings to feel safe and still loved with the arrival of a new baby, and encourages them to feel comfortable, balanced and reassured within the new family set-up.

To accompany all stages of pregnancy, birth and beyond

SAFE PLACE
This spritz offers a sense of peace and tranquillity—a safe place to draw breathe, reconnect with your peaceful centre and move forward feeling grounded and secure. It is also to enhance a feeling of calm in the birthing room. All the family can use this essence.

3. INDEX OF EMOTIONS OR STATES OF MIND

Abundance
Bluebell (AB) promotes universal trust, belief in plenty and joy in sharing.
Harebell re-establishes connection to receiving and success when feeling demoralized.

Addictive behaviour
Forsythia transforms old useless patterns, habits. Helps break addictions.
Milkweed imparts strength, self reliance and healthy ego for demands of normal life.
Urchin helpful in alleviating worry, obsessions and addictions.

Aggression
Balga Blackboy for an overly aggressive or forceful approach.

Anger
Black-Eyed Susan to manage impatience, reduce temper and stress.
Blue Elf Viola to get in touch with and release deep-seated anger and frustration.
Mountain Devil for releasing angry and intense emotions in a more productive manner.
Pink Geranium to release tension and anger constructively and without transferring to others.

Anxiety
Aspen instils safety and security when nervous, uneasy or fearful.

Apathy
Kapok Bush for motivation and incentive if feeling discouraged, exhausted or resigned.

Argumentativeness
Purple and Red Kangaroo Paw for understanding/perspective; diffuses deadlock situations.
Sweetgale to reclaim emotional space and balance after argument or upset.

Arrogance, pride and superiority
Banana replaces self-focus and the need to be right with modesty, humility and dignity.
Vine for encouraging wisdom and understanding. Enhances leadership traits.

Assertiveness
Balga Blackboy for frustration and if forceful because of inability to be assertive.

Authority issues
Red Helmet Orchid tempers a hot-headed or selfish attitude towards those in authority.

Awareness
Birch expands consciousness. Enhances ability to see beyond the self/own concerns.
Lady's Mantle broadens awareness and openness to spiritual perspective.

Balance
Moschatel brings balanced life, fun, enjoyment, self nurturing, fulfilment of one's needs.
Sea Pink for balanced energy flow and awareness of one's highest good.

Bonding
Balsam increases warmth/sensitivity and promotes harmony in relationships.

Wedding Bush for bonding, devotion, commitment and dedication in relationships.

Boundaries
Monkeyflower strengthens one's convictions and certainty, if giving power away.
Monkshood defines strong boundaries and protection when you are wanting to withdraw.

Calmness
Black-Eyed Susan creates balanced inner composure when stressed or hurried.
Hybrid Pink Fairy Orchid helps maintain inner strength and peace.

Caring for others
Alpine Mint Bush for carers who become worn down by the responsibility of others.
Leafless Orchid helps one to know when to stand back and how much to help/give others.
One-Sided Wintergreen deepens one's understanding of how one's energies affect others.
Philotheca encourages one to see oneself as deserving, if giving is over emphasised.

Centring and grounding
Narcissus to feel safe, centred and face challenges without worry.
Pear to remain calm, composed, steady and centred regardless of your circumstances.

Challenges
Thistle for strength, confidence and assurance when overawed by difficulties.

Waratah for staying-power and endurance during difficulties.

Change, coping with
Bauhinia for resistance to new ideas and change.
Bottlebrush for letting go of the past, embracing change, coping with new experiences.
Corn brings renewed mental vitality and the initiative to instigate projects.
Glacier River washes away attachment to what has been before.
Kapok Bush restimulates apathetic feelings and brings a willingness to 'give things a go'.
Letting Go to release self-restriction and limitations.
Poison Hemlock for feeling of being locked in a holding pattern.
Stonecrop helps with inner stillness at times of transformation.
Walnut helps in all transitions and when needing to resist the influence of others.

Changes, resisting
Camellia shifts old behaviour and thought-patterns and self-protective mechanisms.
Lapis Lazuli stimulates communications, energizes the throat area, releases suppresses thoughts.
Pink seaweed releases the past, embraces the 'new'. Increases grounded feeling.
Round-Leaved Sundew when resisting change, identifying too much with the ego.

Commitment
Laurel for strength to put ideas into action without being distracted and giving up.

Sweet Pea for commitment to settle in one place and form bonds with others.

Communication and expression
Bluebell (PAC) if unable to make oneself understood. For speaking one's own truth.
Blue Delphinium enhances listening skills, verbal expression, speaking with integrity.
Catspaw for speaking the truth about hurt feelings, injustices and expectations.
Cosmos for integrating disorganized thought-patterns into articulate speech.
Easter Lily for truth without having to play a role or put on a mask.
Meadow Sage to express strong emotions such as anger without guilt or spite.
Twinflower for listening effectively and communicating from a position of calmness.
Veronica if feeling overlooked/in the background. Brings you out of the shadows.

Conditioning, unhelpful or detrimental
Boab helpful in erasing unhelpful family conditioning and thinking that inhibits growth.

Confidence
Larch encourages confidence and clears patterns of self-doubt or failure.

Conflict, confrontational
Pear reinstates poise, composure and the ability to handle crises.
Macrozamia when quick to respond in an aggressive manner to perceived threats.

Start's Spider Orchid if frustrated, or upset when compromising or avoiding.
Scottish Primrose deals with anxiety, shock, fear, discouragement or quarrelsome states.

Confusion see thinking

Consistency
Peach-Flowered Tea Tree provides consistency to see things through.

Contentment
Pussy Willow encourages sense of own timing, easier to just 'be' rather than always 'do'.

Controlling/manipulative behaviour
Fringed Mantis Orchid for goodwill, kindness, ability to work with best intentions of others.
Grape heals neediness or feelings of abandonment; releases expectations or demands
Isopogon releases bossiness and knowing what is right for others.
Pale Sundew purifies heart, awakens consciousness to controlling, manipulative tactics.

Convalescence, recovery and recuperation
Cotton Grass if holding on to shock and trauma which impedes healing.
Cowkicks re-energizes and rebuilds when exhausted, or going through trauma, accidents, shocks or surgery.
Gorse for strength, faith and renewed hope when feeling hopeless about getting better.
Hornbeam revitalizes mental freshness when tired and weary.

Pink Fountain Triggerplant rejuvenates when depleted by illness, shock or surgery.
Zucchini restores energy and vitality either when ill or during convalescence.

Courage
Dog Rose for bravery and dealing with fear.
Tomato for strength, creating an invincible belief in yourself.

Creativity
Holy Thorn for the ability to share your creativity.
Hooker's Onion creates light-hearted approach which overcomes frustration.
Orange Honeysuckle when frustrated and cannot find outlet for creativity.
Turkey Bush renews confidence in creative abilities.
Wild Iris boosts imagination and inspiration.

Criticism
Fig for self-acceptance. Releases unrealistic, limiting or perfectionist expectations of oneself.
Rock Water for flexibility in excessive self-discipline or denial of your needs.
Sphagnum Moss acceptance to view disappointments in yourself or others not as failures.
Yellow Cowslip Orchid for objectivity, reduces criticism and disapproval of others.

Depression
Cucumber for sadness and detachment. Revitalizes and brings desire to reintegrate into life.
Orange lifts negativity and despair. Renews enthusiasm when apathetic.

Red Rose helps with negative thoughts and finding joy within.
Scotch Broom is elevating when bogged down with pessimism and uncertainty.
Waratah for determination and fortitude if depressed and hopeless.

Despair
Gorse when you think you are never going to recover.
Sweet Hunza to see reason, opportunity and acceptance in challenging situations.

Despondent or downhearted
Chiming Bells brings a feeling of peace and joyful renewal if sad or discouraged.
Gentian to be able to see problems and difficulties without falling into hopelessness.
Lapis Lazuli to dispel despondency and gloom.
Red Grevillea for strength and courage to leave or change uncomfortable situations.
Sunshine Wattle for negativity/pessimism when belief is that difficult times will continue.

Detachment and feeling cut off
Banana to step back, respond calmly, cope without reacting or taking things personally.
Foxglove stops the heart from closing down during/after unpleasant experiences.
Golden Glory Grevillea to cope with other's attitudes without feeling vulnerable
Illawarra Flame Tree for feeling accepted, acknowledged by others. Strong self reliance.

Orange Spiked Pea for a calm expression without reacting intensely.
Physostegia to respond peacefully especially when overwhelmed by forceful personality.
Pixie Mops encourages responsibility for yourself, lessens expectations of others.
Yellow Cowslip Orchid to detach from issues, allowing objective, unbiased, fair appraisal.

Determination
Centaury when doing things to own detriment. Increases individuality and willpower.
Pink Impatiens for courage to stand by own beliefs, determination to do what feel is right.

Dictatorial and domineering behaviour
Gymea Lily brings a modest approach and consideration for others.
Vervain for an open mind, allowing others to have their own opinions.
Willowherb for empowerment. Helps one conduct interactions with humility and diplomacy.
Yellow Leschenaultia for increased sensitivity and understanding of others.

Disappointment
Sphagnum Moss to view disappointments in oneself or others as not necessarily failures.

Discerning/Discrimination
Bladderwort improves discrimination when confused, uncertain or taken advantage of.
Snapdragon raises one's powers of discernment.

Disorganized/undisciplined
Disciple of the Heart brings structure to self or life when muddled or not facing up to things.

Disruptive behaviour
Jasmine when finding it difficult to get on with others. Replaces opposition with diplomacy.

Distant or remote manner
Red and Green Kangaroo Paw encourages being in touch, sharing and attentive.

Ego and personal power
Pineapple for a strong balanced sense of identity and personal power.
Round-leaved Sundew balances ego with wisdom.
Sitka Spruce Pollen for empowering and using your power with good judgment.
Woolly Smokebush for balanced self-importance without being the centre of attention.

Emotions: blocked feelings
Chamomile for stability, emotional objectivity; lessens mood swings.
Flannel Flower for those who are not comfortable with feelings and closeness.
Green Bog Orchid supports healing of issues and blockages held in the heart.
Honesty to express oneself freely; liberates repressed emotions, loosens reserved feelings.
Lettuce for composure and serenity when emotions agitated, or nervous, excitable, troubled.
Mallow unites the mind and heart when feelings are detached from thoughts.

Marie Pavie for confidence to follow inner feelings, good for disappointments.
Moonstone lessens identification with the emotional state, brings control over emotions.
Pink Mulla Mulla heals deep wounds in the psyche, diminishes fear of revealing oneself.
Sitka Burnet for detached emotions, awareness of the real issues to be addressed.
Tall Yellow Top connects the head with the heart, integrating feelings with thinking.
Yellow Cowslip Orchid for people blocked from feelings, too focused in their intellect.

Emotions: intense, agitated or excitable
Banana for when one's judgement is clouded by pride or defensiveness.
Chamomile to calm fluctuating emotions.
Holly transmutes strong feelings like anger and hate.
Indian Pink for centering and calming the emotions.
Lettuce to instil composure and serenity.
Rose Cone Flower for emotional stability when surroundings and circumstances are unsettled.
Scarlet Monkeyflower for facing up to strong emotions, repressed feelings.
Tiger's Eye to distance from emotions if taking things personally.
Tiger Lily tempers hostile attitudes.

Empathy
Yellow Star Tulip imparts sensitivity, compassion, consideration and receptivity.

Empowerment
Dill increases personal power and changes how one is perceived and treated.
Monkey Flower for conviction, boldness, courage and not giving power away.
Rose Alba for taking the initiative and for positive expression of your power and purpose.
Sunflower strengthens you to act in accordance with your full potential.

Endurance see persistence

Energy, overactive
Black-Eyed Susan for slowing down. Calms hyperactivity. Encourages relaxation/inner calm.
Impatiens for slowing down your pace in life.
Purple Enamel Orchid for steady energy, a balance between work and relaxation.
Sponge enables one to relax and maintain peace, transmute other's negative energies.
Stock slows down and balances physical energy.
Verbena for doing too much and being unable to relax.

Energy, depleted, worn out or tired
Aloe Vera for burn-out. Rejuvenating, introducing more balanced energy output.
Kapok Bush for vitality and motivation if incentive and enthusiasm are lacking.
Macrocarpa restores energy and provides endurance at times of challenging activity.
Oak when plodding on with work and becoming more despondent and worn out.
Old Man Banksia restores energy and increases enthusiasm.

Stonecrop for coping with changes without becoming exhausted and listless.
Sycamore uplifts and restores vitality.

Enthusiasm
Passionate Life supplies stimulus and incentive, good for setbacks and obstacles.
Woolly Banksia provides strength, vitality and hope to reach your goals.

Equality
Yellow Hyacinth increases recognition of others if you do not feel equal.

Expanding horizons
Filaree for objectivity, putting life into perspective rather than dwelling on minor problems.
Golden Waitsia to see the bigger picture rather than bogged down with details.
Rabbitbrush to concentrate on a broad vision together with the interrelating parts.

Expectations, letting go of
Hazel frees up controlling, limiting thinking and expectations. Going with the flow.
Letting Go to expand restricting beliefs of oneself. To move forward without limitation.

Expression, see communication

Failure
Sphagnum Moss to avoid seeing disappointment in self or others as failure

Fairness
Swan River Myrtle for victim or perpetrator of injustice.

Fear
Begonia to see life without fear or limitation. Helps to embrace new experiences.

Bog Rosemary to feel safe and protected when immobilized with irrational fears.
Bush Iris for safe awareness of spirituality, eliminates fear of one's psychic abilities.
Grass Widow when embracing a belief system that does not have the support of others.
Grey Spider Flower for calmness during intense fear. Protection against psychic attack.
Lavender when psychically too absorbent or over wrought with spiritual influences.
Mimulus releases fears, brings peace, balance and courage to face the world.
Purple Monkeyflower instils calm when frightened by any aspect of the occult.
Red Clover to perceive events with positivity rather than fear.

Flexibility
Jellyfish encourages a fluid and adaptable attitude.
Wild Rhubarb breaks up stagnant mental patterns, allows the mind to be open to new ideas.

Forgiveness
Dagger Hakea instills lightness, kindness and frees up bitterness, grudges and resentment.
Mountain Devil replaces hatred and anger with acceptance and unconditional love
Rowan for letting go hurts, forgiving self and others.

Frustration
Red Grevillea promotes independence, boldness and help to leave frustrating circumstances.

Fulfilment
Red Huckleberry to find regeneration on a deep level

Groundedness
Fawn Lily for strength to manage everyday affairs. Helps one to utilize spiritual gifts.
Rainbow Glacier for resistance to being in one's body especially after painful experience.
Stitchwort helps sensitive people to feel safe, secure and courage to break new ground.
West Australian Smokebush integrates body and mind when vague and disconnected.

Growth
Spirea works on patterns of resistance; resisting growth by hanging on to old attachments.

Guidance, inner
Cerato brings certainty to believe in own inner guidance.
Viburnum increases intuition, heightens awareness so one trusts in own inner voice.

Harmony
Coral provides skills to live harmoniously and cooperate with others.
Harvest Lily imparts unifying qualities to resolve tension between others.

Hate see forgiveness

Honesty
Easter Lily to express true self without playing a role, putting on a mask or using duplicity.
Fuchsia Grevillea enhances interactions with others that are straight forward and truthful.

Rabbit Orchid releases fear and masks when not being true to self. For openness and truth.

Humility see arrogance

Hurt
Raspberry for reacting touchily, taking things too personally or easily hurt.

Hyperactivity
Almond for self-control, moderation in using time and energy more wisely.
Hops Bush for calm & peace when overstimulated and finding it hard to switch off.

Impatience
Black-Eyed Susan to manage impatience.
Impatiens to increase restraint, patience, tolerance and empathy with others.

Impulsiveness/Impetuousity
Verbena helps create meditative state.

Inadequacy
Pine for blame and guilt. Brings self acceptance/see oneself realistically and deserving.

Inconsistency
Christmas Tree-Kanya for consistency and being comfortable with responsibility.
Strawberry for inner strength and self acceptance resulting in dependable behaviour.

Indecision
Bell Heather restores purpose and direction if undecided and lacking conviction.
Jacaranda brings a quality of focus, which helps to make and stick with decisions.
Lettuce for patience, concentration, calm and decisive thinking.

Pippsissewa dissolves anxiety/confusion around decision making. For empowerment.
Scleranthus brings consistency and reliability when restless, changeable and unfocused.

Independence/individuality
Aquilegia Columbine enhances ability to think and act independently of others.
Buttercup helps relieve need to judge oneself by conventional benchmarks for success.
Happy Wanderer for confidence, self-assurance, independence, self-belief.
Indian Pipe enables you to be involved in a group yet able to express your individuality.
Red Grevillea for frustration of dependence on another. Provides the courage to change.
The Rose for individuality, feeling different or unusual or challenged to express your truth.
Snake Bush to replace needy feelings with self approval and emotional independence.
Walnut if needing to resist the influence of another or to pursue one's own goals.

Inferiority, feeling of
Sea Palm encourages self-acceptance if trying to control everything in life.

Insensitivity
Kangaroo Paw for those that are self-absorbed or totally unaware of others.
Raspberry if reactive and clouded by emotion.

Integrity
Antiseptic Bush for truth to your inner light when compromised/too open to influence of others.

Intimacy
Archduke Charles when putting up barriers. Enhances intimacy, particularly ability to feel safe when touched.
Balsam for warmth, sensuality and sensitivity. Promotes bonding and harmony.
Flannel Flower for sensitivity and gentleness in touching,whether in sexual or sensual way

Intolerance see tolerance

Intuition
Bush Fuchsia to create better balance between creative and logical sides of the brain.

Irritation
Black-Eyed Susan to manage impatience, reduce temper and stress.
Mountain Devil for releasing angry and intense emotions in a more productive manner

Jealousy
Chicory encourages unconditional love if possessive or overprotective.
Mountain Devil decreases jealousy, suspicion and clinging possessively to others.

Joy see also lightheartedness
Illyarrie to face and deal with past traumas, hurts and to re-establish joy in life.
Lily of the Valley to connect with your inner radiance and vitality.
Snowdrop (PAC) for enthusiasm, joy, vivacity and getting moving again.

Lightheartedness, fun, care-free feeling
Fairy Bell lifts feelings of heaviness, increases cheerfulness.
Flannel Flower for carefree and joyful qualities.
Little Flannel Flower helps you express elation and increased enjoyment in life.
Valerian lifts spirits and restores sense of humour.
Zinnia to restore humour, laughter and a child-like playfulness at heart.

Loneliness
Hermit Crab for contentment, peace and coping with loneliness and new environments.
Illawarra Flame Tree thaws out any remoteness or inaccessibility from others.
Lime releases loneliness and overcomes the fear of separation from others.
Red Feather Flower helps one to feel involved and sharing in community life.
Single Delight for connectedness when feeling separate and disconnected from others.
Shooting Star when feeling unwanted, cut off, alienated or not fitting in.
Tall Mulla Mulla when feeling withdrawn or uncomfortable mixing with people.

Love: healing hurts
Bluebell (AB) heals feelings of emptiness and re-establishes trust in sharing with others.
Emerald heals hurts that have blocked further experiences of love.
Pink Cherry helps one to love again after traumatic experience.

Rose Quartz replaces wounds with self love and inner peace.

Love: feeling fearful, needy
Orange Wallflower supplies self love and appreciation.

Love, self-
Alpine Azalea if blocked from feeling love for self or others.
Mauve Melaleuca enhances inner contentment and self-love.
Pink Cherry to fill up an empty, painful heart—unconditional love for oneself and others.

Materialism, excessive concern with possessions and money
Begonia supports letting go of possessions by opening up to trust in the universe.
Bluebell (AB)for universal trust and sharing, a belief in plenty and abundance consciousness.
Bush Iris creates a healthy balance between materialism and other important things in life.
Trillium heals obsessions with the materialism and creates an awareness of spirituality.

Meditation
Aquamarine for a peaceful meditative state and a clear receptive mind.
Cassandra for deep relaxation and stillness of mind open to inner guidance.
Polar Ice to stay quietly in the mind attached only to the present moment.

Mood swings
Chamomile to calm fluctuating emotions and emotional objectivity.

Peach-Flowered Tea Tree when swinging from one extreme to another.
Scleranthus for fluctuating moods and vacillating and wavering thoughts.

Mothering, lack of
Evening Primrose for inadequate mothering/abandonment manifesting as emotional avoidance.
Pink Cherry for warmth and nourishment if experienced insufficient mothering.

Negotiating
Harvest Lily unites/resolves oppositions. Ability to see/appreciate another's point of view.

Nervousness, agitation and restlessness
Almond for moderation, balance if spreading yourself too thinly, resulting in nervous tension.
Coffee stabilizes the nervous system and also reduces the dependence on caffeine.
Comfrey (FES), calms stressed mind, releases tension.
Morning Glory soothes the nervous system and establishes stability in daily routines.

Nurturing, of self and others
Barnacle for those who seek nurturing and nourishment from outside themselves.
Cyclamen honours the needs of the self, especially when exhausted or burnt out.
Goddess Grasstree for balance when under or over nurturing of others
Japanese Magnolia for less dependence on others, self-nurturing, inner fulfilment.

Optimism
Giving Hands to restore hope if exploited, abused or mistreated.
Sunshine Wattle to perceive life differently and to see the future with optimism.
Wild Violet sees things in best light, not missing out through apprehension/pessimism.

Overindulgence
Almond for sexual excesses or over-indulgence in food.
Blue China Orchid for healthier patterns in over-eating/addictions /obsessions. Breaks habits.

Overwhelmed feeling
Elm for overwork or over-responsibility. Removes feelings of inadequacy and doubt.

Panic
Ribbon Pea quells apprehension, foreboding, anxiety and dread.
Rock Rose for ability to cope in overwhelming states, accidents and emergencies.

Past, living in
Hazel shifts resistance to limiting attachments and increases trust in the flow of life.
Honeysuckle for holding on to past, inability to forget events, regret over missed opportunities.
Morning Glory (PF) uneasy circumstances due to living in the past, unwilling to change.

Patience see impatience

Peace
Bluebell Grove provides healing, relaxing, restful, renewing and tranquil inner oasis.
Heart of Peace for balance, proportion, stability. Perceive life with calm detachment.

Lettuce for inner certainty. Nervous excitability replaced by patience and tolerance.
Verbena replaces inner turmoil, rash behaviour and impetuosity with relaxed mind.

Persistence
Coconut boosts energy, increases endurance so barriers are more easily overcome.
Kapok Bush provides persistence to keep going, renews the fighting spirit.
Poppy (Texas) promotes feelings of sharing and involvement with others.

Perspective
Crab Apple to see objectively and in context if stuck in details or petty concerns.
Ox-Eye Daisy for a still, safe, peaceful centre to enable a greater perspective.

Procrastination
Sticky Geranium for lethargy, resistance, indecision and the energy to finish a task.

Protection, from others' thoughts and energy
Daisy shields against overwhelming and turbulent situations and surroundings.
Fringed Violet to protect one from the negative and draining energies of other people.
Guardian for sensitive people. Prevents the absorption of unwanted energies from others.
Hybrid Pink Fairy Cowslip Orchid for inner strength, to be less affected by others.
Leafless Orchid helps one understand exactly how much is healthy to give to others.
One-Sided Wintergreen strengthens energy field, increases sensitivity of others.

Pink Yarrow provides objectivity and detachment for vulnerability to other people.
Yellow Yarrow for protection especially for those who create barriers and close down.

Purpose, direction or guidance
Paper Birch for awareness of which path is in the best interests of whom one really is.
Sapphire for clarity of life-purpose. Aligns spiritual responsibility and capabilities.
Silver Princess supplies guidance if direction is aimless. Inner strength to keep going.
Wild Oat puts one in touch with their purpose and gives direction.
Yellow Dyas connects one's purpose to the larger plan. Good if feeling unsupported.

Quietening the mind and unwanted thoughts
Boronia replaces unwanted, persistent thoughts with stillness and restful sleep.
White Chestnut turns off the internal chatterbox, creating a quiet, calm mind.

Recognition
Cowslip Orchid for feelings of inequality. Brings inner contentment and self respect.

Regeneration
Menzies Banksia brings renewal, rejuvenation and courage to past hurts and pessimism.
Snowdrop (F) replaces dark destructive thoughts with optimism and hope for future.

Rejection
Illawarra Flame Tree for self-reliance if feeling rejected when others not around.

Relationships, break-ups
Black Kangaroo Paw for emotional trauma. Heals hurt, hatred, resentment & anger.
Yellow Pond-Lily for inner security and release of unhealthy emotions or attachments.

Relationships, commitment
Coconut replaces a non-committal attitude with the ability to honour commitments and vows.
Many-Headed Dryandra unites fulfilment with consistent commitment.
Pearly Everlasting instils devotion and fidelity.
Wedding Bush for inconsistency in relationships or trouble in committing to others.

Relationships, dealing with
Australian Bush Relationship to verbalize, express feelings and improve communications.
Bleeding heart unconditional love if possessive. Support at times of brokenheartedness.
Bush Gardenia for loving relationships, ability to convey what you actually feel.
Hematite to maintain independence and strong boundaries within relationship.
Queensland Bottlebrush when using relationships for own benefit.
Start's Spider Orchid to act directly, decisively and with courage and wisdom.
Yellow Pond Lily helps you feel centred despite emotional issues and attachments.

Resentment
Cape Bluebell releases negativity, pain, bitterness. Heals resentment and jealousy.

Donkey Orchid for detachment to walk away from blame and resentment.
Phoenix Rebirth to release judgments of yourself and others and to forgive on a deep level.
Willow brings optimism and awareness of how one's thinking affects one's life.

Resilience
Pink Fairy Orchid instils resilience and calm, unaffected by what is going on externally.

Responsibility
Illawarra Flame Tree encourages responsibility and commitment to course of action.
Red Beak Orchid unites responsibility/duty with desire if unfulfilled desires create frustration.
Ursinia to take responsibility to help others and to work together in common purpose.
Wattle to become aware of reality/face up to things, understand consequences of actions.

Restraint
Almond for self-control, moderation and in using time and energy more wisely.
Vervain instils self discipline and restraint for over-doing or patterns of excess.

Sadness and grief
Menzies Banksia for regeneration, to move through pain into a position of optimism.
River Beauty for cleansing which washes away the hold of powerful emotions.
Sturt Desert Pea to let go of any old hurts and pain which are bottled up or unresolved.

White Spider Orchid encourage spiritual viewpoint and response to life from universal perspective
Yerba Santa for bottled-up feelings. Lightens the heart so emotions flow more freely.

Safety and security
Cow Parsnip for adaptability, stability and feeling at home during changes. Homesickness.
Hermit Crab for contentment, peace and coping with loneliness and new environments.
Honeysuckle for dealing with homesickness, old hurts. Regenerates interest in the 'now'.
Windflower provides one with a sense of self-acceptance and inner security.

Self-acceptance
Agrimony to accept all parts of oneself, take the self more lightly and find peace within.
Alpine Azalea for unconditional self-acceptance and when withholding love from others.
Wild Cyclamen strengthens inner resourcefulness if there is no outside support.

Self-confidence
Larch encourages confidence and clears any patterns of self-doubt and failure.
Snake Vine boosts optimism, belief in oneself, self-worth and confidence in one's abilities.
Tamarack increases self identity and strength in one's abilities during challenging conditions.

Self-control
Vervain lessens over-reaction.

Willowherb for restraint and tact when over bearing or full of self importance.

Self-discipline
Coconut enforces self-discipline and perseverance. Enables one to complete without giving up.
Wandering Jew for discipline and patience. Combines ideas with reasoned thinking.

Self-esteem
Billy Goat Plum if there is dislike of one's physical self.
Five Corners increases self-respect, especially when facing aggressive/competitive behaviour.
Pineapple for contentment with yourself, encourages strong sense of identity
Tamarack to increase self-identity and strength in one's abilities.
Vanilla Leaf instils strong sense of self-approval.
Yellow Cone Flower when feeling undervalued, unappreciated or taken for granted.

Self-responsibility
Lace Flower encourages belief in yourself rather than relying on others for approval.
Pixie Mops to hold yourself in a place of love rather than what you feel others owe.

Self-worth
Gold develops self-esteem and strong sense of identity.
Goldenrod increases self-respect so criticism does not affect one.
Parakeelya encourages self esteem, assertiveness and awareness of one's inner power.
Snake Vine to boost belief in worth of self.

Urchin Dryandra for self-appreciation and self-respect especially if easily exploited.

Selfishness, self-centredness
Cowslip Orchid brings the ability to interact with others on a more equal basis.
Gymea Lily for intolerance, bossiness and domineering qualities.
Heather to encourage approaching life from a less self-centered perspective.
Impatiens to help increase patience, diplomacy and empathy with others.
Kangaroo Paw for being self-absorbed and unaware or insensitive of others.
Lime for focusing on the needs of others rather than just the self.
Peach enhances supportive, caring and nurturing qualities for others.
Spirit Faces (Banjine) encouragement not to see oneself as foremost.
Vine to help recognize that others must also be allowed to reach their own potential.

Sensitivity
Raspberry helps to let things go if taking what others say too personally.

Seriousness
Little Flannel Flower to lighten up and perceive life with more joy.
Poison Hemlock letting go rigid feelings and negativity.
Sea Rocket enhances feelings of security and abundance.

Sexual matters
Macrozamia helps resolve sexual inhibitions or problems such as frigidity and impotence.

Purple Magnolia balances overactive libido or withdrawal from intimacy.

Shock
Pear recover poise and composure when troubled, disturbed, thrown off balance.

Shyness
Violet when shyness means that one feels alone and alienated from others.

Social Consciousness
Quaking Grass find identity through work in groups. Balance own needs.
Sweet Pea conveys feeling of connection with humanity. To find one's own place in society.

Spirituality
Angelsword establishes clear connection with one's higher self.
Icelandic Poppy if hesitant to manifest one's true spiritual identity.
Northern Twayblade helps ground spiritual aspects into physical life.
Urchin for fear of the unknown and when exploring unknown spiritual territory.
White Nymph Waterlily (Miani) encourage spiritual outlook, especially during frustrating times.

Strength
Tomato for strength and stability. Instils courage to tackle known/unknown fears.
Cattail Pollen to project strong sense of self, especially if difficulties and barriers impede.
Pyrite hardens resolve, trust in yourself, ability to stick to decisions and stand up for yourself.

Stubbornness
Bauhinia for resistance to change, obstinate and immovable behaviour in relationships.
Fig increases open minds for over-serious or uncompromising natures.
Isopogon for the tendency to be bossy. Facilitates flexibility and understanding of others.

Stuck feeling
Boab when influenced by inappropriate family values, thinking and traditions.
Jellyfish for a fluid and adaptable attitude.
Honeysuckle for being stuck in past, unable to forget events, regretting opportunities.
Stonecrop for stuckness, resistance and clinging unnecessarily to a view point.

Stress
Black-Eyed Susan to reduce tension, cope with busy situations without becoming stressed.
Bluebell Grove for peace, renewing and healing if stressed and exhausted.
Mint Bush for ability to cope and awareness of spirituality during stressful times.
Purple Flag Flower helps release tension if stressed and under pressure.
Yellow Flag Flower for cheerfulness, seeing good side of life despite pressures or worries.

Submissiveness
Centaury restores individuality and own identity when over-anxious to please others.

Support
One-Sided Bottle Brush when feeling alone, unsupported, overwhelmed by demands.
Pink Impatiens for strength if overwhelmed, unsupported or coping with challenges.

Tact and diplomacy
Purple Eremophila for diplomatic skills. Separating emotions from the issues at hand.

Thinking, assimilation
Paw Paw to make decisions and digest new information and ideas without being overwhelmed.

Thinking, clarity, focus and concentration
Blue Lupin simplifies issues, releases anger, brings focus to confusion.
Brown Kelp to look within without fear, confusion or relying on old survival patterns.
Broom stimulates mental clarity, concentration and integration of thoughts.
Bunchberry reduces distraction and being sidetracked. Fosters concentration and mental clarity.
Clematis for dreamy, inattention, indifference, unrealistic or confused states.
Lettuce essence for calm, clear, concentrated thoughts.
Pink Trumpet Flower focuses the mind to enable completion of tasks.
Sundew to stay focused in the real world, instead of mentally absent or in a dream.
Yellow Boronia for overactive, scattered mind, unfocussed thinking and distraction.

Thinking, fixed
Blackberry for positive thinking rather than narrow, picky or negative.
Dampiera promotes flexibility, accommodation and adaptability.
Isopogon for when one thinks one is one is always right.
Pincushion Hakea for encouraging a discriminating yet practical view of things.
Wild Rhubarb breaks up stagnant mental patterns, opens to new plans, ideas and solutions.

Thinking, hyperactivity
Nasturtium restores vitality when continual mental hyperactivity is exhausting.
Yellow Boronia to concentrate, focus and calm and soothe mental activity.

Thinking, improving memory
Avocado (MA) for alertness, attentive to details and improved memory function.

Thinking, negativity
Azurite expands consciousness enabling beliefs and negativity to be refreshed.
Crab Apple is cleansing and purifying when stuck in details or negativity.
Iona Pennywort for when issues to confront, dark or denied thoughts to face up to.

Thinking, overly rational
Hibbertia integrates intuition and rationality so thinking is more flexible and less narrow.
Lamb's Quarters for when one understanding is limited by being too rational.
Shasta Daisy for more complete integration of ideas rather than just analytically.

'Staghorn' Algae, to perceive from a higher perspective particularly if mental turmoil.

Thinking, over-serious thinking
Little Flannel Flower to lighten up and trust that life can be enjoyed.
Freshwater Mangrove opens one to new opportunities and ideas, releases intolerance, prejudice.

Thinking, repeating mistakes
Isopogon if not learning from mistakes or experiences.

Thinking, scattered
Jacaranda for a clear head and focus on achieving tasks.

Thinking, unwanted thoughts
Lettuce for control of thought-processes, rather than letting them run wild.
White Chestnut turns off constant thoughts and creates a calm quiet mind.

Tolerance
Banana for qualities of humility and objectivity
Beech when always seeing wrong in a situation or others. For being judgmental.

Date for an open mind and receptiveness to others if intolerant and unaccepting.
Red Quince for not reacting defensively.
Slender Rice Flower for flexibility to listen to others.
Yellow and Green Kangaroo Paw for understanding. Reduces sharp appraisal of others.

Understanding
Raspberry to encourage understanding and be less affected by emotion.

Unpredictability
Peach-Flowered Tea Tree for unpredictable energy or fluctuating from one extreme to another.

Victim consciousness, see also empowerment
Geraldton Wax for standing own guard, not easily influenced or compromised by others.
Lobelia for strong boundaries if easily influenced by others. Can say 'no' if you want.
Parakeelya for self-esteem, assertiveness and inner power if feeling 'like a doormat'.
Southern Cross for optimism if creating a victim consciousness through negativity.

Vulnerability
Grass of Parnassus brings serenity to face hurt and sadness. Lifts the spirit.

Will
Apple for self-discipline, inner strength and the right use of will.

Wisdom
Hairy Yellow Pea to step back from anxiety and worry before making a decision.
Scots Pine helps inner listening, enhances intuitive powers, increases inner certainty.

Workaholic
Orchid, dancing lady for contentment if working to compensate for perceived failures.
Moschatel when thinking life has to be hard and to achieve comes with great effort.
Vervain for any patterns of overdoing or overwork.

Worry
Crowea for calmness if coping with stressed, worried, troubled or anxious states.
Spinach for seeing life simply, without complication and with humour.

4. PRODUCERS OF ESSENCES

Initials at head of entry are those used in the main text and in the lists

AB
Australian Bush Flower Essences
45 Booralie Road
Terrey Hills
NSW 2084
Australia
Tel: +61 2 9450 1388
www.ausflowers.com.au
info@ausflowers.com.au

AL
Living Essences of Australian Flowers
11/59 Walters Drive
Herdsman Lake
W.Australia 6017
Australia
Tel: +61 8 9443 5600
www.livingessences.com.au
email@livingessences.com.au

ASK
Alaskan Essences Inc
PO Box 1090
Victor
MT 59875
USA
Tel: +1 406 642 3670
www.alaskanessences.com
afep@ alaskanessences.com

B
Healing Herbs Ltd
PO Box 65
Hereford
HR2 0UW
England
Tel: +44 (0) 1873 890 218
www.healingherbs.co.uk
info@healingherbs.co.uk
or from
The Dr Edward Bach Centre
Mount Vernon
Sotwell
Wallingford
Oxon
OX10 0PZ
Tel: +44 (0) 1491 834 678
Fax: +44 (0) 1491 825 022
www.bachcentre.com
mail@bachcentre.com

F
Findhorn Flower Essences
Cullerne House
Findhorn
Moray
Scotland
IV36 3YY
Tel: +44 (0) 1329 690129
www.findhornessences.com
info@findhornessences.com

FES
Flower Essence Services
PO Box 1769
Nevada City
CA 95959
USA
Tel: +1 530 265 9163
www.fesflowers.com
orders@fesflowers.cokm

GEM
PHI Essences BV
Rijksweg Zuid 1
NL 5951
AM Belfield
Tel : +31 (0) 77 475 4252
www.PHIessences.com
info@PHIessences.com

LH
Light Heart Flower Essences
PO Box 35
Halesworth
Suffolk
IP19 0WL
Tel: +44 (0) 1986 789 168
www.lightheartessences.
co.uk
info@lightheartessences.
co.uk

SN
Spirit-in-Nature Essences
14618 Tyler Foote Road
Nevada City
CA 95959
USA
Tel: +1 530 478 7655
www.Spirit-in-Nature.com
info@Spirit-in-Nature.com

PAC
Pacific Essences
Box 8317
Victoria, BC
V8W ER9
Canada
Tel: +1 250 384 5560
www.pacificessences.com
info@pacificessences.com

PER
Perelandra Ltd
P.O. Box 3603
Warrenton
VA 20188
USA
Tel: +1 540 937 2153
www.perelandra-ltd.com
email@perelandra-ltd.com

PF
Petite Fleur Essences Inc
PO Box 330411
Fort Worth
TX 76134
USA
Tel: +1 817 293 5410
www.aromahealthtexas.com
petitefl@aromahealthtexas.
com

5. ESSENCE DISTRIBUTORS

This list gives UK distributors only. In any case of difficulty, contact the producer for a list of suppliers

ESSENCE WORLD
94 High Street
Eton
Berkshire
SL4 6AF
England
Tel: +44 (0) 1753 863214
www.essenceworld.com
helpme.now@essenceworld.com

FLOWER SENSE LTD
19 London End
Beaconsfield
Buckinghamshire
HP9 2HN
England
Tel: +44 (0) 1494 671775
www.flowersense.co.uk
info@flowersense.co.uk

HEALTHLINES
The Barn
Town Yeat
Underbarrow
Cumbria
LA8 8DN
Tel: +44 (0) 1539 68761
www.healthlines.co.uk
admin@healthlines.co.uk

INTERNATIONAL
FLOWER ESSENCE
REPERTOIRE
Achamore House
Isle of Gigha
Argyll & Bute
Scotland PA41 7AD
Tel: +44 (0) 1583 505 385
www.healingflowers.com
flower@atlas.co.uk

NATURE'S WISDOM
Unit 10c Dabble Duck
Industrial Estate
Shildon
Durham
DL4 2RA
England
Tel: +44 (0) 1388 778197
www.natureswisdom.co.uk

NELSON BACH
Nelsons House
83 Parkside
Wimbledon
London
SW19 5LP
Tel: +44 (0) 20 8780 4200
Fax: +44 (0) 20 8789 0141
www.nelsons.net
enquiries@nelsons.net

PANOSUN LTD (PER)
The Lockenburg Centre
10 St Leonards Road
Forres
IV36 1DW
England
Tel: +44 (0) 8454 308 607
www.panosun.org
info@panosun.org

THE ESSENCE SHOP
Tel: +44 (0) 1264 365450
+44 (0) 1264 850176
Online only
www.theessenceshop.co.uk

UNIVERSAL ESSENCES
Tel: +44 (0) 870 062206
www.universalessences.com
essences@universalessences.com

6. INDEX OF ESSENCES

AGRIMONY (B)
Almond (SN)
Aloe Vera (FES)
Alpine Azalea (ASK)
Alpine Mint Bush (AB)
Angelsword (AB)
Antiseptic Bush (AL)
Apple (F)
Apricot (FES)*
Archduke Charles (PF)
Aquamarine (ASK)
Aquilegia Columbine (PF)
Aspen (B)
Australian Bush Rel'ship (AB)
Avocado (FES)*
Avocado (SN)
Azurite (ASK)

BABIES' BREATH (PF)
Bachelor's Button (PF)
Balga Blackboy (AL)
Balsam (F)
Bamboo (PF)
Banana (SN)
Barnacle (PAC)
Basil (PF)
Bauhinia (AB)
Beech (B)
Begonia (PF)
Bell Heather (F)
Billy Goat Plum (AB)
Birch (F)
Blackberry (SN)
Black-Eyed Susan (AB)
Black Kangaroo Paw (AB)
Black Mushroom (PF)
Bladderwort (ASK)
Bleeding Heart (FES)
Bluebell (AB)
Bluebell (PAC)
Bluebell Grove (LH)
Blue China Orchid (AL)
Blue Delphinium (LH)
Blue Elf Viola (ASK)
Blue Lupin (PAC)
Boab (AB)
Bog Rosemary (ASK)

Boronia (AB)
Bottlebrush (AB)
Broccoli (PER)
Broom (F)
Brown Kelp (PAC)
Bunchberry (ASK)
Bush Fuchsia (AB)
Bush Gardenia (AB)
Bush Iris (AB)
Buttercup (FES)

CAMELLIA (PAC)
Candystick (PAC)
Cape Bluebell (AL)
Carrot (PF)
Cassandra (ASK)
Catspaw (AL)
Cattail Pollen (ASK)
Cecil Brunner (PF)
Centaury (B)
Cerato (B)
Chamomile (FES)
Cherokee Rose (PF)
Chicory (B)
Christmas Tree-Kanya (AL)
Chiming Bells (ASK)
Chiton (PAC)
Clematis (B)
Coconut (SN)
Coffee (FES)*
Comfrey (FES)*
Comfrey (LH)
Coral (PAC)
Corn (SN)
Cosmos (FES)*
Cotton Grass (ASK)
Cowkicks (AL)
Cow Parsnip (ASK)
Cowslip Orchid (AL)
Crab Apple (B)
Crowea (AB)
Cucumber (PER)
Cyclamen (LH)

DAGGER HAKEA (AB)
Daisy (F)
Dampiera (AL)
Dandelion (FES)

Date (SN)
Dianthus (PF)
Dill (PER)
Disciple of the Heart (LH)
Divine Being (LH)
Donkey Orchid (AL)
Dog Rose (AB)

EASTER LILY (PAC)
Elm (B)
Emerald (ASK)
Eucalyptus (FES)*
Evening Primrose (FES)

FAIRY BELL (PAC)
Fawn Lily (FES)
Fig (SN)
Filaree (FES)
Fireweed (ASK)
Fireweed (PAC)
Five Corners (AB)
Five Flower Remedy (B)
Flannel Flower (AB)
Forsythia (PAC)
Foxglove (ASK)
Freshwater Mangrove (AB)
Fringed Lily Twiner (AL)
Fringed Mantis Orchid (AL)
Fringed Violet (AB)
Fuchsia Grevillea (AL)

GAILLARDIA (PF)
Garden Mum (PF)
Gentian (B)
Geraldton Wax (AL)
Giving Hands (AL)
Glacier River (ASK)
Goddess Grasstree (AL)
Gold (ASK)
Goldenrod (LH)
Golden Glory Grevillea (AL)
Golden Waitsia (AL)
Gorse (B)
Grape (SN)
Grass of Parnassus (F)
Grass Widow (PAC)
Green Bog Orchid (ASK)
Green Rose (FES)*

Grey Spider Flower (AB)
Guardian (ASK)
Gymea Lily (AB)

HAIRY YELLOW PEA (AL)
Happy Wanderer (AL)
Harebell (F)
Harvest Lily (PAC)
Hazel (F)
Heart of Peace (LH)
Heather (B)
Hematite (ASK)
Hermit Crab (PAC)
Hibbertia (AB)
Holly (B)
Holy Thorn (F)
Honesty (LH)
Honeysuckle (B)
Hooker's Onion (PAC)
Hops Bush (AL)
Hornbeam (B)
Hybrid Pink Fairy/
   Cowslip Orchid (AL)

ICELANDIC POPPY (ASK)
Illawarra Flame Tree (AB)
Illyarrie (AL)
Iona Pennywort (F)
Impatiens (B)
Indian Pink (FES)
Indian Pipe (PAC)
Iris (PF)
Isopogon (AB)

JACARANDA (AB)
Japanese Magnolia (PF)
Jasmine (PF)
Jellyfish (PAC)

KANGAROO PAW (AB)
Kapok Bush (AB)

LACE FLOWER (ASK)
Lady's Mantle (F)
Lamb's Quarters (ASK)
Lapis Lazuli (ASK)
Larch (B)
Laurel (F)
Lavender (FES)
Leafless Orchid (AL)
Letting Go (LH)

Lettuce (SN)
Lily of the Valley (PAC)
Lime (F)
Lobelia (PF)
Little Flannel Flower (AB)

MACROCARPA (AB)
Macrozamia (AL)
Magnolia (PF)
Mallow (FES)
Many-Headed Dryandra (AL)
Marie Pavie (PF)
Mauve Melaleuca (AL)
Meadow Sage (PF)
Menzies Banksia (AL)
Milkweed (FES)
Mimulus (B)
Mint Bush (AB)
Monkey Flower (F)
Monkshood (ASK)
Moonstone (ASK)
Morning Glory (FES)
Moschatel (ASK)
Moss Rose (PF)
Mountain Devil (AB)
Mountain Wormwood (ASK)
Mulla Mulla (AB)
Mussel (PAC)

NARCISSUS (PAC)
Nasturtium (PER)
Northern Twayblade (ASK)

OAK (B)
Old Man Banksia (AB)
One Sided Bottlebrush (AL)
One-Sided Wintergreen (ASK)
Opal (ASK)
Opium Poppy (ASK)
Orange (SN)
Orange Honeysuckle (PAC)
Orange Leschenaultia (AL)
Orange Spiked Pea (AL)
Orange Wallflower (LH)
Orchid 'Dancing Lady' (PF)
Ox-Eye Daisy (PAC)

PALE SUNDEW (AL)
Paper Birch (ASK)
Parakeelya (AL)
Passionate Life (LH)

Paw Paw (AB)
Peaceful Detachment (LH)
Peach (SN)
Peach-Flowered Tea Tree (AB)
Pear (SN)
Pearly Everlasting (PAC)
Peppermint (PF)
Philotheca (AB)
Phoenix Rebirth (LH)
Physostegia (LH)
Pincushion Hakea (AL)
Pine (B)
Pineapple (SN)
Pink Cherry (LH)
Pink Fairy Orchid (AL)
Pink Geranium (PF)
Pink Impatiens (AL)
Pink Mulla Mulla (AB)
Pink Seaweed (PAC)
Pink Trumpet Flower (AL)
Pink Yarrow (FES)
Pipsissewa (PAC)
Pixie Mops (AL)
Plantain (PAC)
Poison Hemlock (PAC)
Polar Ice (ASK)
Polyanthus (PAC)
Pomegranate (FES)
Poppy (Texas) (PF)
Purple/Red Kangaroo Paw (AL)
Purple Enamel Orchid (AL)
Purple Eremophila (AL)
Purple Flag Flower (AL)
Purple Magnolia (PAC)
Purple Monkeyflower (FES)
Pussy Willow (LH)
Pyrite (ASK)

QUAKING GRASS (FES)
Queensland Bottlebrush (AL)

RABBITBRUSH (FES)
Rabbit Orchid (AL)
Rainbow Glacier (ASK)
Ranunculus (PF)
Raspberry (SN)
Red/Green Kangaroo Paw (AL)
Red Beak Orchid (AL)
Red Carnation (PF)
Red Chestnut (B)

Red Clover (LH)
Red Feather Flower (AL)
Red Grevillea (AB)
Red Helmet Orchid (AB)
Red Huckleberry (PAC)
Red Leschenaultia (AL)
Red Quince (LH)
Red Rose (PF)
Revelation (F)
Ribbon Pea (AL)
River Beauty (ASK)
Rock Rose (B)
Rock Water (B)
Rough Bluebell (AB)
Round-Leaved Sundew (ASK)
Rose Alba (F)
Rose Cone Flower (AL)
Rose Quartz (GEM)
Rowan (F)
Ruby (GEM)

SAGUARO (FES)
Salmonberry (PAC)
Salvia (PF)
Sand Dollar (PAC)
Sapphire (ASK)
Scarlet Monkeyflower (FES)
Scheranthus (B)
Scotch Broom (F)
Scots Pine (F)
Scottish Primrose (F)
Sea Horse (PAC)
Sea Lettuce (PAC)
Sea Palm (PAC)
Sea Pink (F)
Sea Rocket (F)
Shasta Daisy (FES)*
She Oak (AB)
Shooting Star (FES)
Single Delight (ASK)
Silver (ASK)
Silverweed (F)
Silver Lace (PF)
Silver Princess (AB)
Sitka Burnet (ASK)
Sitka Spruce Pollen (ASK)
Slender Rice Flower (AB)
Snake Bush (AL)
Snake Vine (AL)
Snapdragon (PF)

Snowdrop (F)
Snowdrop (PAC)
Soapwort (PF)
Southern Cross (AB)
Sphagnum Moss (ASK)
Speedwell (LH)
Spike Lavender (PF)
Spinach (SN)
Spinifex (AB)
Spirea (ASK)
Spirit Faces (Banjine) (AL)
Sponge (PAC)
'Staghorn' Algae (PAC)
Starfish (PAC)
Start's Spider Orchid (AL)
Sticky Geranium (ASK)
Stitchwort (LH)
Strawberry (SN)
Stock (PF)
Stonecrop (F)
Sturt Desert Pea (AB)
Sturt Desert Rose (AB)
Sundew (AB)
Sunflower (FES)
Sunshine Wattle (AB)
Surfgrass (PAC)
Swan River Myrtle (AL)
Sweetgale (ASK)
Sweet Hunza (LH)
Sweet Pea (FES)
Sycamore (F)

TALL MULLA MULLA (AB)
Tall Yellow Top (AB)
Tansy (PF)
Tamarack (ASK)
The Rose (LH)
Thistle (F)
Tiger's Eye (ASK)
Tiger Lily (FES)
Tomato (SN)
Trillium (FES)
True Power (LH)
Turkey Bush (AB)
Turquoise (ASK)
Twinflower (ASK)

URCHIN (PAC)
Urchin Dryandra (AL)
Ursinia (AL)

VALERIAN (F)
Vanilla (PF)
Vanilla Leaf (PAC)
Verbena (PF)
Veronica (AL)
Vervain (B)
Viburnum (PAC)
Vine (B)
Violet (FES)

WALNUT (B)
Wandering Jew (PF)
Waratah (AB)
Watermelon (FES)*
Water Violet (B)
Wattle (AL)
West Austr. Smokebush (AL)
Wedding Bush (AB)
White Chestnut (B)
White Nymph Waterlily
  (Miani) (AL)
White Spider Orchid (AL)
Wild Cyclamen (LH)
Wild Iris (ASK)
Wild Oat (B)
Wild Oats (PF)
Wild Pansy (F)
Wild Violet (AL)
Willow (H)
Willowherb (F)
Windflower (PAC)
Woolly Smokebush (AL)

YELLOW BORONIA (AL)
Yellow Cone Flower (AL)
Yellow Cowslip Orchid (AB)
Yellow Dryas (ASK)
Yellow Flag Flower (AL)
Yellow Hyacinth (LH)
Yellow Leschenaultia (AL)
Yellow Pond-Lily (PAC)

ZINNIA (FES)

* Essences whose properties
  are still being researched.